Wh

"Lynda Hébert has written a must-read wellness guide for anyone wanting to be the best version of themselves. It's an absolute game changer, transforming you from the inside out. This book isn't just a book to read, it's a book to be practiced."

— Dena Pope Jordan, Blue Diamond Leader
Wellness Advocate
Forsyth, GA

"Lynda offers specific skills that help you live life to the fullest, with a holistic approach to thriving in body, mind and spirit. What follows is a reflection of a passionate life message that when fully embraced means, not guilt-induced, but joyful transformation. I love it and you will too."

— Beth Hendley, Lifelong Church Community
Developer, Individual and Family Counselor
Wexford, PA

"Lynda's knowledge, heart and passion shine in every written word of this book. Her genuine desire to empower others to radically and confidently own their health and wellbeing soaks through these written pages and speaks straight to the heart. The guidance she provides, when applied, can be life altering for generations to come!"

— Tamazeen Barber, CEO, Livin Alōha LLC
Nokomis, FL

If you'd like to find out more about living Strong, Sane & Sassy, please visit the author's website at www.LyndaHebert.com.

STRONG, SANE & *SASSY*

EIGHT PROVEN POWERFUL LIFESTYLE HABITS THAT TRANSFORM YOU FROM THE INSIDE OUT

Lynda Hébert, BSN

BrightLife Publishing

Strong, Sane & Sassy
by Lynda Hébert

LyndaHebert.com

Published by BrightLife Publishing

ISBN: 979-8-9900547-0-7 (paperback)
ISBN: 979-8-9900547-1-4 (eBook)
Cover & Book Design by Nick Zelinger, NZGraphics.com

Disclaimer:
Although the author and publisher have made every effort to ensure the accuracy and completeness of information contained in this book, we assume no responsibility for errors, inaccuracies, omissions, or any inconsistency herein. Any slights of people, places, or organizations are unintentional.

Your use of the information in this book does not create a doctor-patient or other professional relationship between you and the author or publisher. The information shared in this book is not meant to diagnose, heal, or treat any disease.

First Edition

Printed in the United States of America

To Diane, my late beloved big sister,
and to Ricky, my late adored little brother,
This book was born from my heart of love for you.
Through your story and these pages, I hope to help
others develop the same sense of true health and
wellness that I so desperately wanted for you.

Always in my heart,
Your sister Lynda

Table of Contents

1 This One's for You

Welcome, I am thrilled that you are here! By selecting this book you're stepping into a life-changing journey towards authentic health and lasting wellness. My deepest hope is that this book empowers you to live *your* healthiest life possible, rooted in your deepest beliefs from the core of your being. This is not a linear path; it is an intentional journey of personal growth and learning. Your destination is to fully immerse yourself in a highly empowering, yet simple wellness lifestyle.

To be more precise, you are headed toward thriving in foundational, sustainable wellbeing, and I'm eager to walk this path beside you through these pages. My excitement is palpable as I picture your energy levels climbing and intensifying day by day.

Now, it may take some time for you to get to the point of eagerness and vigor that I experience nearly every day. But that's okay! This is a journey, a process. Time isn't only necessary here – it's welcome. So, savor every minute of it.

To get things started, I have a question for you: Are you *thriving* in your wellbeing, or just *surviving* in it? To best answer that question, look at your day-to-day life.

- Are you experiencing life with steady energy and vitality?
- Are you living most of your days refreshed and pain free?
- More often than not, do you feel a sense of anticipation as you embrace the challenges of your day?
- Are you engaging in your routine with a clear, focused mind?
- Are you going about your day trusting and knowing your body can function optimally doing what you want it to do for you?
- Are you living most days fulfilling your purpose with joy?

Maybe you're someone who deeply thrives on the quality of health you experience and the vitality of life that comes with it; you have ambitious personal goals, and you know you need help to support your body, mind, and spirit in the best possible way. Or …

- Do you notice an energy slump by midday, but push through it anyway?
- Are you struggling with headaches, backaches, or fatigue?
- Does your digestive system feel out of sorts, or does your metabolism feel sluggish and underactive?
- Do you notice you're fighting off colds and viruses frequently?

- Are you carrying around anxious thoughts almost like it's normal, or having mood swings and not knowing why?
- Are you lugging around extra weight, and /or burdens that aren't yours to carry, but you do it anyway?
- Do you ever find yourself frustrated, discouraged, or overwhelmed about certain parts of your health and wellbeing?

If your day-to-day life sounds more like the second description than the first, here's the next question to consider:

How long have you been ignoring that inner voice that's aching to be heard?

You know the one: It's gently nudging you, telling you you're neglecting parts of yourself that need attention and nourishment, and that you're taking your amazing self for granted. It's trying to warn you that you're compromising your inner truth and integrity. It won't pipe down about how you're just making choices that are "good enough" instead of choices that are in alignment with your true authentic self.

If that sounds like you, don't worry. Most of us live this way, going through life disconnected from parts of ourselves, without even acknowledging it. I used to wrestle often with feeling like an "imposter." I was too busy to slow down to listen inwardly, and somewhere deep inside, I knew it. And I'll share more on that important matter later. However, for now – even if you've been living in low energy and ignoring that true voice inside – I have some great news for you.

You *can* live your life with steady energy and vitality. I know you may not believe me right now, but I've been there, right where you are, struggling to keep up with life's demands, and unsure if I could ever truly change … until I pushed past that doubt with a new belief. And, just like me, you can change – right where you are. You are not too busy, not too messy, not too complicated, not too young, not too old, not too … whatever story you are telling yourself. You can do it. I know you can! It's very much within your grasp.

And that's why I wrote this book: To make that more possible for ***you.***

By reading this book, you are saying YES to a healthier you. And if you question whether to give yourself permission, like I once did, here's the answer to that question: Yes, *you are so worth it.*

What you are creating is a step-by-step plan for better habits that will give you thriving health and wellbeing not for days or weeks, but for a *lifetime*. My deepest hope is that these habits become a lifestyle manual for you. The goal of your habits is to internalize them, as they automatically become first and foremost who you are, not just what you do. You are going to be establishing these integrated, holistic, healthy habits, and who you will *become in the process* is the best part. You might even feel like doing cartwheels with all the invigorating energy you experience, and you'll thrive living in truth and freedom from the depths of your being.

If you take my words and experiences to heart, then I'm confident in reassuring you that you'll become an empowered owner of your health and wellbeing. I will connect with you, and in turn, you will connect with yourself so that these life-giving concepts incorporate into your lifestyle habits. You will love being integrated with your mind, body, and spirit as you live authentically healthy in your whole being.

But as with anything that seems too good to be true (even when it's not!), as you look ahead at the journey to come, doubts may start sneaking in like uninvited ants at a picnic. And again, I say: That's okay! We all struggle with self-doubt and fears of failing. I've certainly wrestled with these intruding thoughts when I commit to a new goal. Even right now, permeating the excitement I feel as I write this book, there's a voice creeping up behind me whispering, "Are you sure you have what it takes to write this book? Do you really think your message can make any difference?" Oh yes, these disturbing doubts do come and go, yet, having just a seed of faith, joining forces with loved ones, and listening to a supportive voice can help you move forward in confidence. Even if that voice comes from the pages of a book like this one.

So, remember, you are not alone. We are on this journey together. You've got this; I know you do! As well, we need to remember we each have our own unique journey, so in a world of constant comparison, we need to not compare our progress or success with others. Because as you take each step, over time, you'll be amazed by how far you're going. I'm confident in that because when I look back on my own health journey, I see so much transformation.

How It all Started

I'm transitioning now, exposing parts of my story I buried in shame for quite some time. My journey started many years ago, unknowingly, as I witnessed my siblings' health struggles.

In my early teenage years, I watched in agony as my sister Diane and her mental health completely unraveled. As a result, so did her life. Diane was my big sister and best friend, we were inseparable, until her personality started to change. Everything about her became unpredictable from her moods to her habits. She'd swing from being angry with me for no apparent reason to suddenly acting like her normal self. I found myself feeling intensely anxious and confused around her, unsure of what each day would bring. I painfully struggled to make any sense of it all. What's happening to my sister? How do I help her? Those two questions raced through my mind day after day. I was deeply afraid of losing her, and I was also afraid *of* her. She was diagnosed with chronic schizophrenia, and my heart and life felt as if shattered into a million pieces. Over time, all attempts to help her live a healthy life failed. This long season of suffering felt unbearable, as the sister I once knew no longer existed.

Not long after that, my younger brother Ricky who seemed healthy and well, developed a drug addiction that wreaked havoc on his body, mind, and soul. I vividly remember my shock and disbelief over watching what he was going through, and how helpless I felt – again.

He fought hard to recover, focusing on his military career and law school, as my parents and I battled beside him. But when he received the disheartening news: He had developed lymphatic leukemia, he spiraled downward. Aggressive treatment – including a transplant of my own bone marrow – kept him alive for only a short season. I had ferociously prayed and prayed for God to save him, hoping my transplanted marrow would be what he needed to recover. Instead, his journey and death left me feeling completely exhausted and numb.

I desperately wanted my brother and sister to get back on a healthier path. I stuck by them through every medical treatment, but it all proved unsuccessful. I begged God to heal them. He didn't. It was a devastating season of life for me as I tried to work through the grief of losing them both (my sister to chronic psychosis). As a mother with young children, there wasn't much space to fully mourn. Seasons of hurt and anger asking, "Why, God?" were followed by feeling sad and guilty about not finding a way to restore my siblings' health.

Yet in time, as I poured out my anguished soul, God compassionately led me to a place of trust. I felt safe being honest and vulnerable with Him. Eventually, that intimacy molded my identity. I knew who I was: His daughter, fully known and deeply loved. God held me close and held me together during the storm that never seemed to let up. I became resilient.

Experiencing my siblings' destructive lifestyle choices and debilitating health ignited a blazing fire within me to discover true whole health. As a result, I found myself with an unquenchable thirst to understand the root cause of unstable health. This consuming desire drove me to search for answers and solutions. And when I set my course for Ohio State University to earn a nursing degree, my passion intensified.

As I studied and listened to my professors, I soaked in the absolute beauty of each vital organ and efficiently high-powered system in our body. I gained an overwhelming wealth of knowledge about how brilliantly designed, incredibly intelligent, and truly interconnected our entire body is. I became awed by the human body from the inside out. Graduating from Ohio State and working in various settings and fields stimulated my desire even more to understand the body's true healing processes.

However, in time, working as a nurse left me disillusioned about the sick-care model that dominated our healthcare system. Of course, I deeply respected my medical colleagues and thrived on seeing patients recover following surgical procedures and was grateful for the value of medicine. But I didn't understand why so many pills were used to correct symptoms, while the root cause of the problem often went entirely ignored. Why were food, exercise, and other lifestyle habits not addressed? Why were so many people not taught to understand the powerful connection between their own body with their own actions and the tremendous impact this has on their health. I was confused and bewildered.

Something. Wasn't. Right.

I began relentlessly seeking ways to support root level health. I had a desire to live in a real, naturally healthy state, and having children only intensified that desire, because I wanted it for them as much as I wanted it for myself. I knew there had to be better answers out there, so my pursuit persisted.

Season after season, I explored ways of creating and sustaining foundational health. With new experiences and endless research, step-by-step I cultivated an empowering holistic health-oriented lifestyle. Feeling deeply satisfied and extremely hopeful, I developed the confidence to take ownership of my own health.

My brother's and sister's stories continue to impact me like a cascading waterfall, but instead of drowning me, they usher in new life. The scars from that season are the most beautiful parts of me now. Through my suffering, a greater purpose was born. I came to understand that life is not just a senseless mess. God breathes life into our dead dreams and resurrects them. The story is never really over.

I now realize that the dominating thoughts we choose to think, what we believe, the emotions we consistently feel, the types of food we choose to eat, how much water we drink, how often we move our body, the quality of our rest and sleep, and how we interact relationally with others all become our lifestyle habits. And these lifestyle habits become the health we live in, shaping our very wellbeing. And when we are intentional with these habits, we give ourselves the power to be foundationally healthy, producing strength and vitality, from the inside out.

In the scientific research I share throughout this book, you will come to see that certain lifestyle habits we choose create a significant risk in developing sickness and disease.

But more importantly, *our lifestyle habits can also give us the power to prevent and, in some cases, reduce that sickness and disease.* I share this proven fact to empower you and to give you hope.

Maybe right now you don't even know your lifestyle habits. That's okay, because like me, your awareness will grow, and your desire will, too. *Strong, Sane, and Sassy* will guide you to develop these intentional yet simple lifestyle habits that keep *you physically resilient, crystal-clear minded, and true to your own voice and values.* So, no matter where you are or at what age and stage in life you may be, these lifestyle habits will make an enormous difference in your health and wellbeing.

The choices each woman (and man) makes now, whether you're thirteen, thirty-five, or sixty-nine years old, from the quality of your thoughts to the quality of your diet, have the power to ensure vibrant health and wellbeing for the rest of your life. Please let this truth soak into every cell of your being!

The ache in my heart for Diane and Ricky drove me to discover and develop true life-giving holistic healthy habits.

With my whole heart, I believe I was put on this beautiful planet to share my knowledge and passion for holistic health, and my deep appreciation for the human body, mind, heart, and spirit. I want to empower you (and myself) to live as truth-oriented, energy-loving, naturally based health-minded women (and men)! We can't outsource our health to anyone else, so we must engage in it ourselves.

Oh, and yes, my cellular-level, health-nerd side will go all scientific at times throughout this book, but please have patience with me! Because once you see how magnificently God made our bodies from the microscopic level on up, you won't help but love the science of it all just as much as I do.

We can't outsource our health to anyone else, so we must engage in it ourselves.

Living Strong, Sane, and Sassy Through Lifestyle Habits

As I have traversed life, I've come to realize that in some seasons, it's relatively easy to treat my body well, while in other seasons, it's strikingly more challenging. As women our seasons shift and change often, sometimes without warning, and we must adjust to them. For example, we might experience the onset of pregnancy, a friend or family member moving away, a child developing new needs, an unexpected diagnosis, our workplace downsizing, suddenly developing allergies, a loved one spiraling into an addiction … the list goes on. Like a car suddenly rear-ending us, a new challenge can fall upon us and shift our trajectory. That's why having healthy, tried and true, sustainable habits in our lives is foundational. They keep us physically strong, clear-minded, and true to our own values – no matter what befalls us.

In other words, our healthy habits cultivate and solidify us to live strong, sane, and sassy – all in the very best of ways! *Establishing these healthy habits is key to transforming your wellbeing, so that instead of just surviving, you're flourishing!*

This is the first element in this book I encourage you to highlight, underline, circle, or do whatever it is that makes you come back to reread it and meditate on it:

These simple yet powerful habits bring about incremental changes (not a "quick fix") that over time lead to true, lasting change in your wellbeing and your lifestyle, resulting in a new sense of identity, as an authentically healthy, strong-spirited, integrated woman or man.

The intention of this book is to teach you about those habits, why they're important, and how you can implement them into your personal lifestyle.

But before we can even dive into those habits, we need to set some extremely important baselines for you to build them from. Because without a solid foundation, the walls and roof of a house have no chance of standing strong over the decades. Just the same way, when it comes to healthy habits, you want them to last forever.

There are two important foundations to explore before getting to your habits:

- Anchoring yourself in your core beliefs/values
- Aligning your actions with your core beliefs/values

Anchoring yourself in your beliefs/values begins with the courage to dig deep and recognize those things that you want to build your life on. For example, one of my core beliefs is that God loves me and His love for me never changes. My conviction in God's unchanging love gives me a solid base for making decisions about how I interact with myself and others and helps me stay true to my values. Holding to your unshakable beliefs is crucial, giving you the strength to continue thriving in challenging times. Standing on your beliefs and your firm foundational truths fosters confidence and stability in any season of life.

Aligning your actions with your core beliefs/values is the next step. You can identify your beliefs/values all day, but if you don't act on them, then they must not really be your values or what you really believe. What you invest your time and energy in reflects what's most important to you. For example, I deeply value my relationships with my children and grandchildren. Some of the actions I do regularly that align with that core value are scheduling time to be with them, being available for them, and playing with them. I also value personal growth, for myself and for others. That is why I developed habits and rhythms in my day/week for writing, reading, building friendships, holistic health coaching, teaching yoga, exercising outside, enjoying nutritious food, learning new things, and adventuring. Living your days in what you value the most brings true health, joy, and freedom.

It's important to revisit your personal values as new seasons come and go. Some of your values may change as higher priorities crystalize for you. Change is a divinely designed healthy dynamic, especially for women, even though we resist it sometimes. It can be exciting, and somewhat daunting, to uncover hidden desires and be awakened to new callings arising within us. When we give ourselves freedom to do this, our souls thrive. Reassessing helps us to stay on this path of healthy, truthful living.

After you've anchored yourself in your beliefs and aligned your actions with your core values, it's time to get to the habits you'll develop. And to identify those, we're going to walk in STRENGTH.

STRENGTH represents eight sustainable, tried and true, healthy habits that we learn to carry within us every day. This book will unpack this powerful acrostic so you can learn how to specifically implement and integrate these holistic habits into your lifestyle:

Supportive Listening: Sense your Body's Signals
Train Your Thought Patterns
Rest and Rejuvenate
Exercise and Move
Nutrify and Hydrate
Goal-Set with Grace
Thrive in Your Community
Hone Your Healthy Habits

As we go chapter by chapter exploring STRENGTH, we will dive into:

- **How to *truly* support your body, mind, and soul.** You'll discover your core needs by listening to your body's physical sensations, deciphering its signals, and asking yourself clarifying questions.

- **How to establish healthy resources.** You'll learn pertinent knowledge, effective mindsets, skillsets, and toolsets that are readily accessible to you.

When you start to feel achy, stressed, or fatigued you'll have healthy support to turn to instead of resorting to mindless eating, anxiety flare-ups, or an energy crash.

- **How to renew and replenish yourself.** You will come alive as you develop routines of deep breathing and establish lifegiving rhythms of rest in your day-to-day life. You'll learn ways to richly rest, thoroughly replenish, and restoratively sleep.
- **How to incorporate movement into your daily life.** You'll love movement and what it does for you – more than you could ever imagine! Think: oiled joints, a healthy heart, strong muscles, a well-run digestive system, a robust metabolism, flowing energy, and a happy mind.
- **How to tap into the power of nutrition.** You'll come to appreciate the gift of food, and the physical energy and mental boost we gain from what God designed our magnificent bodies to eat and absorb. You'll learn to love food and enjoy it – mindfully. You'll eat in a way that your body naturally reaches your ideal weight. And you'll recognize the tiniest indicator of dehydration approaching so you can savor every drop of life-giving H_2O you consume.
- **How to properly set goals that are achievable and motiving.** You'll adopt the mindset to value the process of working toward your goals instead of just

fixating solely on the end result. It's about who you are becoming throughout the process!

- **How to value and prioritize true community.** You'll learn how community positively impacts your wellbeing. This will lead you to strengthen your current connections and seek out new ones.
- **How to hone powerful, healthy habits.** You will take everything you learn and adapt it to your lifestyle, becoming habitually healthy.

In time and with practice, you will carry STRENGTH in your mind, body, and spirit so naturally that you won't know any other way to live! These practices will help you walk through life confidently and truthfully as you intentionally live out your unique purpose, all the while owning your personal health and wellbeing.

Now, are you ready to roll up your sleeves and get started living in STRENGTH?

Let's go!

2

Preparing to Live in STRENGTH

Your Vision, Your Will, and Your Why

This might be surprising to you, but you and I visualize all throughout our day. That's because when you imagine your future life or a potential future outcome to a scenario, you're visualizing. "Imagining the future" is the simplest way to explain what it means to visualize. It is a mental process we all inherently do.

We visualize what we might be eating for dinner, and we visualize the new house that we hope to buy one day. Ambitious young dancers visualize performing on a big stage. Sales executives mentally rehearse important sales pitches before giving them to potential customers. However, many people spend more time visualizing what they don't want (their fears) instead of their hopes and dreams.

Though you may be visualizing throughout your day, you may not be doing it *with intention,* and that's what you'll be learning to do.

The Power of Visualization

Would you start a race if it didn't have a finish line? Such a scenario would likely lead to immense exhaustion and discouragement! There would surely come a moment in the race when your uncertainty about the endpoint would make you just give up.

Visualization is a way of imagining the finish line. You might be wondering how this relates to our journey to thriving in health. Well, our brains tend to fulfill their most dominant thought. When we visualize, our brain's visual cortex is activated, which causes neurons to fire and creates an internal simulation or mental image that can help us plan and execute future actions based on that simulation (Kosslynn and Thompson, 2006). Research indicates that the subconscious mind cannot distinguish between a real event and one that is vividly imagined (Ram, 2022). Isn't that incredible – *we have the power to experience what we visualize.* So, if we visualize the healthiest version of ourselves, not only are our brains and minds moving in that direction, but so are our bodies and spirits.

Visualization is a way of imagining the finish line.

By God's perfect design, a vision keeps your mind on the future goal and helps you see, feel, and believe what you're working to establish before it's manifested in your life. This is why I'm a believer in creating an intentional vision that you revisit frequently.

Several studies have been conducted on the power of visualization on athletes and how it can improve their performance. One such study by the Cleveland Clinic asked one group of adults to lift weights for 15 minutes a day, five days a week. A second group was asked to perform the same weightlifting program, but to do so while visualizing the muscles they were working on. Over the course of six weeks, the results showed that visualizing muscle growth increased the participants' strength by about 30 percent. On the other hand, the regular group only had an 11 percent increase. (*The Science Behind Visualization and Muscle Growth: A Study –* Selfpause.com). What an amazing example of the mind-body connection.

It seems that the most effective way to expand your potential is to constantly expose your mind to a multi-sensory image of the result you're striving for. This image then serves as a command to the brain to reproduce outwardly what was created inwardly (Newberry, 2007). So, if you deliberately feed your mind clear, vivid pictures of the person you want to become, that energy has the potential to propel you toward your target like a rocket!

Create Your Wellness Vision

Let's take advantage of how your mind works by cultivating what I call your *Wellness Vision.*

Begin by brainstorming all the positive possibilities of living in the best health you could ever imagine. Think forward one, three, or five years from now and imagine yourself truly healthy in mind, body, and spirit.

The most important questions to ask yourself are:

- **What do I want?** Be bone-level honest with yourself about your truest desires. This is for you, and your unique life. Remember, don't let those inner voices of doubt shove down what you really want. Hold nothing back! Then, think about yourself achieving those dreams and ask:
- **What do I see?** If you took a picture of your life, what would be in the picture? Now, really focus on that picture and ask yourself:
- **What am I doing, and how do I feel?** Are you power walking, running, or biking? Do you feel the sweat on your back, the gentle breeze blowing on your face? Do you hear your feet hitting the trail and your puffy breath? Are you and your spouse, and maybe your children, streaming down snow-covered slopes on skis? Can you sense your quadricep muscles engaging as you turn? Are you joyfully engaged with your children or grandchildren, and able to get up from the floor with ease? During your daily routines, are you in a flowing rhythm? Do you have steady, productive energy as you navigate your children's developmental needs, and/or as you run your business? Are you savoring quiet times of rest and renewal that recharge your body and soul? Are you doing what you love?

- **Where am I, and how do I feel?** Are you enjoying the first moments you awaken and arise with ease and anticipation? Are you feeling the freshness of a new morning while doing a yoga routine? Are you gathered around the dinner table with your family enjoying the conversation while mindfully enjoying your flavorful food? After your meal, as you stride along your favorite path with your spouse and/or your children, is your body internally energized from the satisfying, powerful nutrition?
- **How do I look, and how do I feel?** Is your skin smooth and soft? What is the expression on your face? Peaceful, content? How is your posture? Do you carry yourself (and your babies and toddlers) with confidence – engaging your core and back? Do you move with ease and energy?

Now that you have a clear vision of your future, think about how it would be brighter if you made changes to reach that optimal, healthy woman (or man) you see yourself being. Then focus on it deeply. How could making a change in one area of your life improve the rest of it? How could this change benefit your family, relationships, finances, and career path? What positive shifts would you be able to see in your near future?

Now, revisit this vision often! Start off your morning routine with your Wellness Vision or set aside a few minutes in the middle of your day for it. You'll be amazed by how quickly your mind begins to see and do what you feed it. I encourage you to approach this process intentionally to train your mind. See yourself fully alive physically, emotionally, mentally, and spiritually, loving what your body does for you and the overflowing positive impact you have on the people around you.

Here's how I often approach visualization: First, I take some slow, deep breaths and imagine that I'm completely free of false opinions, fears, or negativity of any kind. If I need to, I jot down my fears. Then, I connect with God, acknowledging His presence and His power as He's guiding me, prompting me to visualize specifically, to move beyond my fears and toward my hopes, convictions, and faith-filled dreams.

Visualization is actually one of my favorite activities in my quiet time by myself. I love using my mind and my senses to "see" and "feel" those exact fervent hopes become a reality in my life and in those I love.

I'm excited for you to discover how consistently holding onto the images of what you believe God wants for you makes those images much more likely to become a reality.

Make a Vision Board

A vision board is exactly what it sounds like: A board decorated with visual representations of what you desire most for your life. A vision board can help you hold onto your Wellness Vision and to focus on it daily. You've already done the hardest part by answering the above questions. Now let's go to the fun part and be creative!

First, find pictures, graphics, words, and symbols that reflect the future health and wellbeing you desire. You can cut pictures and words out of magazines or find graphics and images online. You could also use old photos or other objects around your home.

For example, maybe an attractive bike could reflect your energy, agility, and freedom. Or some aerobic running shoes might symbolize your goal to run or walk a mile or enter a 5K or a 10K. You might use an airplane taking off to call out your adventurous spirit, or a serene mountain lake indicating your calm inner spirit. Other ideas include finding facial expressions and bold words that reflect the future health you yearn for.

Once you have all your images ready, find a two-by-two-foot corkboard or magnetic board and arrange each picture onto it in an eye-catching collage by stapling, thumb tacking, or magnetically placing it on your vision board. And, *voila!* You've now created your unique health and wellness vision board! Place it somewhere you'll see it every single day, such as propped up on your bedroom dresser or hanging on the wall in your home or workplace office. Extra points if it can be the very first thing you see when you wake up, and the last thing you see before falling asleep.

What makes your vision board powerful is that it reflects your personality, your values, and your God-given gifts, along with what makes you feel alive, healthy, and well! Your wellness vision board doesn't necessarily have to be anything grandiose, just something that is truly reflective of the authentic wellbeing you desire.

Let me share a couple of tips with you at this point. First, when attempting to create something new in my life, I've learned that I need to make new space for it. I've come to realize that simplifying and decluttering everything in my environment and in my head, including social media, sets me up with a sense of freedom. I now have the space for these new visions and lifestyle habits to grow and flourish.

Second, personal growth involves change, and change can be uncomfortable. Frustration or weariness can creep in when you're on your way to something new and different. That's why it's important to hold on to your vision. Remember that "every great work, every big accomplishment, has been brought into manifestation through holding to the vision" (Shinn, 2010).

Examine Yourself

The previous sections were all about examining your hopes for the future. Now, we'll move into questions to help you clarify where you are right now, a process that involves self-examination and reflection on your habits.

The ancient Greeks saw the wisdom of this process. In fact, Socrates thought reflection was so important that he said, "The unexamined life is not worth living" (Plato's "Apology").

Reflection involves stepping back to examine our present reality. Tommy Newberry, a *New York Times* best-selling author and life coach, has said, "To advance forward, we must retreat" (Newberry, 2007). On this journey of true health, it's important to do this before beginning our journey, and to incorporate rhythms of retreat as needed. We want to get to an honest place and not hide anything, so we can openly and freely move forward in an authentic way. I find this does wonders for my soul.

Are You Willing to Change?

I encourage you to open your mind and heart, along with a journal, and jot down some of your thoughts about your habits. Remember to notice and affirm your profitable habits as well. Also remember that none of us do well when we feel judged or shamed either by ourselves or someone else. I know from experience that we can be our own worst critic. So please don't judge yourself. Instead, show yourself compassion and affirm yourself with every discovery you make about your choices and habits.

To guide you in this process, ask yourself the following questions, and answer honestly and without judgment:

- Am I willing to slow down and take inventory of myself – my true self?
- Am I willing to get to the root cause of my low energy?
- Will I take note of my personal habits and notice which ones are truly supporting me and which ones are distracting or disempowering my wellbeing?
- Am I willing to examine how I spend my time, maybe by recording what I do each hour of my day?

- Will I look at the use of my time and how it does or doesn't keep me on the path to good health or reflect my true voice, core beliefs, and values?
- Without judgment, am I willing to stop eating when I'm full, chew more, and take time to enjoy all the flavors and textures of what I'm eating?
- Am I willing to start a new way of mindful, intentional eating that energizes my body and sharpens my brain?
- Do I make the time to move my body in enjoyable ways?
- Am I ready to honestly examine the stress in my life that leads me to make poor choices like worrying, undereating, overeating, isolating myself, working too much, or not staying true to my core values?
- How do I sleep? What is my regular routine every night in the hour leading up to bedtime?
- How much water do I drink every day?
- Am I willing to carve out time to rest in order to listen to my body's needs?
- Am I ready to accept that I am completely responsible for my own health?
- Will I seek additional support when I need it?

Whew! Sometimes asking yourself the hard questions and facing your truthful answers is the only way to live in complete freedom and become truly healthy. This process in itself is hugely productive. Being honest with yourself about where you are is the main point of this exercise. In addition, this process of asking/answering hard questions honestly with yourself helps you see where you are in relation to your core beliefs/values and identify where you need to change.

From my own experience, facing the truth is the catalyst that changes destructive and disempowering habits. I remember nine months after my third child was born, I found myself escaping twice a day, sometimes three times, to our neighborhood convenience store, dashing in to get an ice-filled Big Gulp of Diet Coke. I got an immediate kick from the caffeine, and it became my go-to coping mechanism when I felt my energy tank depleting. It spiraled into more than a craving; it was an addiction I couldn't function without. A giant Diet Coke started my morning, carried me through my afternoon, and ended my day.

I deceived myself by ignoring my body's signals warning me of the toxic effects that so many chemicals were having on me. I hurt my adrenal glands, overstimulated my brain, and deprived my kidneys of the water they needed to function well. I felt conflicted, because I knew something wasn't right, but I couldn't stop.

However, once I took the time to truly consider and draw upon my core value of inward integrity, I came to grips with this addiction and what that drink was actually doing to my body. It was a destructive habit that took me a long time to overcome, but I eventually did it.

I will say, battling that bad habit with young children at home was quite difficult. So, if you're in a similar situation, please understand this truth: When you make any beneficial change in your own life, you make your children's lives better, too. So, instead of thinking, *I don't have the time to invest in my own wellbeing right now,* consider shifting your thinking to: *I **must** invest in my own wellbeing and make it a priority, so my children will value their own wellbeing as a priority, too.* In addition, your children will undoubtedly thrive with a well-balanced, naturally energized mom.

As we wrap up the topic of examining yourself and facing the habits you want to change, it's vitally important to understand that changing ultimately comes down to a *decision of your will.* If you are genuinely wanting *and willing* to change, and you ask God to help you persevere, then you are well on your way.

We'll close this chapter with one more way to prepare to live in STRENGTH.

Know Your Why

What is your "Why?" It's your internal motivation, your driving purpose for changing. Your *why* will keep you moving on your pathway, focusing on the specific road to flourishing in STRENGTH. Your *why* helps you stay on the gas when you feel like slowing down, turning back, or throwing on the brakes.

First, discover and pinpoint your why, and then get clarity on it. Consider these questions:

- Why did I pick up this book?
- Why do I want to begin this journey?

- Why do I want to reach this goal? Further questions to this end could be:
    - Do I want to approach each day with a full tank of energy?
    - Do I want to live pain-free?
    - Do I want to sleep soundly and wake up with energy and excitement for the new day?
    - Do I want to carry a peaceful spirit within myself?
    - Do I want consistent joy?
    - Do I want to live life at my natural weight for my body?
    - Do I want to be a vibrant and stronger mom?
    - Do I want to run my business with productive energy and clear focus?
    - Is something about my health holding me back from my highest calling and passion?
    - Do I want to show up more truthfully and authentically for myself?
    - Do I want to finally tap deeper into the specific talents and gifts I was designed with? To live out that creative spirit within me and make a difference in all the lives around me?
    - What dream have I planned and visualized, but never taken action on?

Remember, get clear on your *why* (and it's okay to have more than one). Ask God to help you in this journey. He will, beyond your imagination! He's helped me more than I could have ever dreamed.

Keep working on your *why.* No one's health and wellbeing are one-size-fits-all. Know your *why* and revisit it when you need greater clarity, focus, and motivation. Continue sharpening and refining it as you grow.

It's with great pleasure that I say you are now prepared to begin your journey to true health by learning to live in STRENGTH! Now that you are in better tune with who you are and who you wish to become, you are ready to approach this path with clarity, courage, and commitment, anticipating the thriving health you will feel in every season to come.

Let's take a look at the S in STRENGTH.

3 STRENGTH

Supportive Listening: Sense Your Body's Signals

Yes, here we are at our exciting entrance into unpacking STRENGTH! And it starts with establishing a solid foundational habit that transforms you from the inside out. It's a habit that allows you to thoroughly sense what your body is telling you, and deeply search your soul. And this habit is called *supportive listening – a valuable strategy to sense your body's signals.*

What is supportive listening? It's investing your time to listen to someone with genuine interest and devoted attention, while probing for understanding, meaning, and clarity. In this case, the someone is YOU. The goal of supportively listening is to gain true understanding of the needs and desires of someone you love. And this is precisely the depth of listening we want to apply as *we learn to listen inwardly – to ourselves!*

Part 1: Listening Inwardly to Yourself

Have you considered if you really listen to yourself? Listening to yourself in a way that's healthy and productive starts with slowing down. And that isn't always easy. But when you do, you can pinpoint where your inner signals are coming from. Once you identify that, probe them further for better understanding and clarity. This is at the heart of listening to yourself – knowing what your mind, body, and heart are trying to communicate. It involves focusing on all those cues and signals that you may have trained yourself to overlook and ignore for quite some time.

And listening to yourself is where true health begins. After all, you're the only one who experiences your body's sensations, thinks your thoughts, and feels your emotions. No one else can do that for you (though there are some who might like to try). As you learn how to listen to yourself, you'll understand more clearly what you need and want at your deepest level. You then become your wisest friend and most effective healthcare provider.

But learning to hear your body's signals takes time. If you've been drowning out your voice for most of your life, it will take a while to tap into that inner knowledge. Throughout this process you must be willing to tap into your own intuition.

Unfortunately, we've learned how to tune out our body's signals. I know this through my own experience. My body constantly tried to tell me what it needed, but I couldn't hear it. Instead, I was too busy telling *it* what to do. I often ignored the feedback it gave me. I had believed pushing past my own signals was the best way to carry on.

Personally, my story of hushing my inner voice started early in life, and it's taken me time to retrain myself to listen inwardly. It began when I was four years old, playing kickball in the backyard with my sister and our neighbors. It was my sister's team's turn to kick and run the bases, and I was the pitcher. But I vividly remember feeling tired and wanted to be done playing (as four-year-olds are prone to do), so I dropped the ball and headed for the back door of the house.

My sister ran after me, pushed me to the ground, and jumped on my chest. To this day, I distinctly remember the crushing feeling of her weight on me and gasping for air. I felt overwhelmed and shocked. That experience, I believe, taught me to silence my desires and opinions not only to my sister, but to others and to myself.

I also recall a physical trainer at a local gym instructing me in lifting weights. I knew something was off because my back felt compromised. Yet I stayed silent, ignored the strain my back was experiencing, and continued to lift. As a result, my back wasn't the same for quite some time.

As time passed and my search for true health intensified, I awakened to the value of my own body's messages. I made the commitment to myself to do the work of reflection and examination inwardly, and I gained insight into myself. Through God's divine help, I found the courage to get downright honest with myself.

I got to the root problem; I discovered I was living fragmented, disconnected, not in unity with myself. My body, mind, and heart were not integrated, and I was ignoring significant parts of myself. My eyes were opened to my lack of integrity. That exposure drove me to clear out my old ways and begin new habits of creating and establishing *true* wellness and wholeness from the inside out.

I started eagerly teaching myself to recognize my body's internal sensations, and then to process the signals my heart and my gut were telling me, such as my feelings of disappointment, uneasiness and anger.

As I learned and practiced supportive listening, I discovered even more! Living this way brings freedom, builds tremendous confidence, and deepens my respect for my body – and for the One who designed me. And I am thrilled to tell you that I finally gave up the dance of shallow listening. I developed an authentic inner relationship with all parts of myself.

And I love living this way!

I now tune in to clearly understand the cues and messages of my body, mind, and heart. The voices I listen to have now changed. What I "should" do, think, and say no longer drive my choices. I honestly listen with curiosity, going past the fear of what I might face, accepting my body right where it is, and the condition of my soul. As I respond to my body's informative signals and acknowledge what I'm feeling inside, my sense of personal ownership has grown.

And the best part is – this changed deepened my relationship with myself, with God, and with others, as I became more truthfully me. As a result, my health and wellbeing improved dramatically.

Developing this genuine relationship with myself did not happen overnight – I'm still working on this new way, and I sometimes return to my old well-traveled path, especially when stress creeps in. Curiosity and compassion help me find my way back to the healthy way, as I acknowledge where I am without judgment. So don't be discouraged if it happens to you, too. The reality is that you may have spent most of your life unaware of what your body is trying to tell you, so now it's going to take time to really listen to your God-given true self and learn to hear and express your own authentic voice. And I'd like to add one other note and here it is: Living by our own made-up (or someone else's) unspoken rules or expectations derails you from listening inwardly at your core level of health.

Your voice reflects your God-given identity to the world around you. That divinely formed unique voice inside of you is yours only, as well as your own God designed biology. I've learned it's important to acknowledge it, develop it, and freely flourish in it (and it all starts with supportive listening). Then, who you are on the inside and the outside will be united, living in integrity throughout your entire being, without hiding or shaming any part of yourself. You will experience truth "in the inward being," and "wisdom in the secret heart" (Psalm 51:6 ESV). Yes, nothing beats this way of living!

Your voice reflects your God-given identity to the world around you.

When we begin forming a new habit, *time and repetition* are necessary for the change to become automatic, and learning to listen to yourself is no different. And that's our goal during every step of STRENGTH: creating new habits that, over time, replace old habits.

You are going to hear your body tell you things you've never imagined. You are going to find inner confidence that you never knew existed. All of this is coming to you because you are showing up truthfully! In the rest of this chapter, you will learn how to sense your body's communication signals, interpret its very own language, and respond in nurturing ways with effective natural solutions. Your goal here is to learn to identify what you need and want both at a cellular level and within your deepest inner being.

Supportive listening is the heart of true health, so this chapter will be your foundational heavy weight for living in STRENGTH.

Part 2: Sensing Your Physical Body Signals

The body functions as a whole, and we need to listen to every part of it to support its needs as a whole. But to truly live this way, we must first understand the most seemingly simple concept of our entire wellbeing: A single cell holds the key to the whole organism.

Our cellular level is the root of all our wellbeing, and it's also the root of all our sickness, injury, and disease. How? Because single cells come together to form tissues, and tissues come together to form organs and glands. Therefore, keeping individual cells healthy is the only way to experience health in the whole body. In other words, to thrive is to feel well at a foundational level in your microscopic cells.

To keep our bodies healthy, we need to identify two essential things when we listen to our physical bodies:

- What do the cells of my body love?
- What do the cells of my body detest?

Now remember, we are unique people who are as different on the inside as we are on the outside. Your body knows how to get you well, so you just need to listen to it and support it in that endeavor! Let that sink in and give you a true sense of empowerment. Once you embrace this process, *you* get to help yourself heal from the inside out. I like to refer to this as your personal "cell care."

And embracing this process first means understanding how it works. Yes, that means we are going to dive into some magnificent, intelligent science about the human body!

The Central Nervous System

Our central nervous system is truly an incredible thing because it helps keep us alive by using two parts that work in harmony—the sympathetic nervous system and the parasympathetic nervous system. Understanding your central nervous system and the way it interacts with you is important, because it consistently gives you feedback on how your thoughts, actions, and reactions affect your body and your sense of wellbeing.

The sympathetic nervous system oversees your body's "fight or flight" response. When it senses danger, the sympathetic nervous system floods your body with hormones that make your heartbeat faster, your breath quicken, and your muscles tighten. These are the preparations your body needs to make so that you can effectively choose whether you will fight the danger at hand or flee from it.

Your parasympathetic nervous system helps you maintain homeostasis, which is the state of steady internal body conditions. Your parasympathetic nervous system helps you to recover from the effects brought on by the sympathetic nervous system and allows your body to rest, digest, and recover. Our cells love spending a majority of their life in a parasympathetic state. It's where our bodies are most comfortable, where they get to restore and repair and keep things functioning at their best.

But when some kind of stress signals your body to fight or flight, your adrenals begin pumping cortisol. Then your body immediately responds by speeding up blood flow to your heart, so you can prepare to run or fight. Because so much energy is put into this process, at the same time, things like your digestive system, reproductive system, and other bodily systems slow down until the stress has passed. Only when your body feels "safe" again do your adrenals stop pumping cortisol, so your central nervous system returns to a parasympathetic state and gets to work on healing and repairing what your cells need to reenter homeostasis.

With me so far? Good!

Now, here's the kicker: If your body continues to receive stress signals that instigate fight or flight, it will continue pumping cortisol. And that's one of the biggest problems we humans are all facing these days. We experience so many stresses in life, whether they're truly life-threatening or comparatively minuscule, that our bodies can experience a near constant sympathetic nervous system state. Or, if it's not constant, it's at least occurring much more often than our biological systems were designed for it to happen.

Remember, some other important processes in our body like our reproductive, digestive, and immune system are halting, waiting for our body to return to a parasympathetic state. And that waiting can create imbalances like decreasing our hormonal production or keeping our immune system from becoming stronger.

Our cells are glad to receive extra support when danger is truly near, but when they are consistently overstimulated with cortisol, inflammation surrounds them, and they become unhappy and weak. We become more susceptible to viruses, panic attacks, fatigue, insomnia, and digestive problems. In addition, exposure to too much stress, a poor diet, or inadequate sleep and rest creates more damage in our cells over time. After just a few years of living in chronic stress, our bodies can begin to break down. We find ourselves with conditions like lupus, rheumatoid arthritis, thyroid imbalances, adrenal fatigue, low energy, a poor immune system, unexplained weight gain, and other hormonal imbalances that disrupt our reproductive system and our metabolic processes. The National Agriculture Safety Database has even estimated that as much as 90 percent of illness and diseases like high blood pressure, cardiovascular disease, and type 2 diabetes are stress-related (Thames and Thomason, 1997).

Please hear me now ... if you are experiencing symptoms of one or more of these conditions, *you did not cause it!* There are numerous variables involved when stress creeps into our life. It's often unexpected and unannounced and in many ways something that we cannot control. *However, the point to remember and to practice is this:* Identify your body signals of stress and recognize what those signals are telling you and then learn to support yourself with intentional habits that reduces and relieves that stress.

As you can see, the overall goal then is to move yourself in and out of the sympathetic nervous system state and parasympathetic nervous system state with ease, and to generally spend most of your time in the parasympathetic nervous system state. But the problem is, life isn't stress free. Part of living includes experiencing all the little daily stressors that can build up into stormy seasons. You may not even realize when your sympathetic nervous system is kicking in to protect you from stress, because you've gotten so used to feeling that way so often. You might think you have a handle on your stress, but it may very well be handling you!

Recognizing that and taking the power back to change these stressful elements in your life is fundamental to moving forward. Thankfully, your body is good at telling you when it's experiencing stress *and* at giving you clues about how to alleviate it. So, if you can effectively learn to identify your internal and external stressors, and respond with support, you can remain in a parasympathetic state instead of moving into fight or flight unnecessarily.

Of course, there will certainly be times when you absolutely do need to fire on all cylinders, like when you're running after your three-year-old who darted out into heavy traffic; then, it's imperative that your body jolt you to act fast and think quickly so you can protect your child. That type of fight or flight response might be necessary once a week, every other day, or sometimes multiple times a day if you have a particularly rambunctious three-year-old!

But, when you begin to feel fight or flight symptoms when it seems like there's no true reason for them, this is something to pay very close attention to. If there's no danger or need to react quickly, but you feel your heart beating faster, the muscles in your body tighten, or your breath getting shallow and quick, it could be that you're developing anxiety regarding a situation in your life. Maybe you're dwelling, ruminating, or obsessing over your thoughts so much that your body is reacting in hyper vigilance as a way of staying alert to what it perceives as danger. As a result, our frontal lobes, where we think, reason, and organize, then become frazzled, and we can no longer think rationally or sensibly. "No one gets smarter under stress," says Charles Morgan, a forensic psychiatrist at the University of New Haven in Connecticut, in an article from *NewScientist* (Bond, 2017).

Listening to your body and your inner truth can help you manage this stress. Looking at your responses to real and imagined stress is an eye-opening practice. But how, exactly, do you do that?

Show Up for Yourself

First, connect with your breath, focusing your mind on inhaling and exhaling. When you learn how to slow down your thoughts by connecting with your physical body and focus on your breathing, you will relax and regain composure.

Next, pay attention and clearly sense your body's signals in these moments. Show up with compassion and curiosity about your wellbeing by focusing on what you're experiencing physically, along with examining your thoughts and emotions when that stress reaction arises. You can take out your journal, or just sit with yourself, and take a moment to slow down and ask yourself these questions:

- What am I experiencing right now:
  - Physically? Do I have any tight muscles, digestive upset, a tension headache, shallow breathing, or a fluttering heart?
  - Mentally? Am I having difficulty focusing, experiencing scattered thinking, or a sense of mental overload?
  - Emotionally? Am I feeling anxious, fearful, or a general sense of uneasiness?
- What has caused me to feel this way?
- What do I know to be true about the situation?
- What do I need to change in my thoughts and my emotions surrounding the situation?

The goal here is to understand and listen within. Once you've identified what you're feeling and what it is that's making you feel that way, you have the power to reduce that perceived stress, make the necessary changes, and re-anchor yourself in truth.

And then, you can address your body's needs. For example, you can soothe tight muscles with some stretching, or rest your tired mind by doing something fun and playful.

For me, sometimes stress comes from intrapersonal conflict. When this happens, I feel the blood rushing out of my head and my arms, and I sense myself becoming uneasy and alarmed. Once I calm my inner emotions, think through what has happened, and get a clearer perspective, my thoughts and my emotions begin to shift.

And in time, extending compassion and/or forgiveness to myself, or maybe my husband, restores me, grounds me, and re-anchors me in truth. Because of that, sometimes I spontaneously break out dancing to music in my kitchen with my husband or grandchildren! They love it—and my para-sympathetic nervous system loves it too! Or I may participate in hugging for an entire twenty seconds. Yes, research shows that hugs can reduce stress by boosting the release of hormones in our bodies that prevent the sympathetic nervous system from staying activated (SCL Health, 2018). How about that?

Eventually, this process of reducing the time you spend in your sympathetic nervous system state will get easier and more natural to do. And your less-stressed cells will thank you!

As we progress through STRENGTH, and you learn these mindsets, skillsets, and toolsets, you can actually buffer the matrix of your body (the connective tissue that surrounds all the cells and organs of the body) from high cortisol. Living and flowing between your sympathetic nervous system to your parasympathetic nervous system will become a natural dance for you. And living mostly in your parasympathetic nervous system state will become a way of life for you.

The Digestive System

Your digestive system speaks to you more than any other system in your body because of its powerful impact on your mind.

Wait a minute, did you read that right? You sure did! I'll say it again: Your gut health is directly related to your mental health.

Decades ago, when my sister was struggling with poor mental health, looking anywhere but the brain for an answer was inconceivable to medical professionals. Now, science shows just how much of our brain's mental health is related to the food we eat and our stress levels. And the gut is a good place to start when trying to get to the root problem of a mental health disorder.

For my sister and her health team, her lifestyle choices were never addressed. But boy do I wish I had known back then that what she was eating was a key factor preventing her from getting better. Mountains of processed foods and sugary snacks kept her brain in a fog. Her diet didn't help her sleep, and contributed to her anxiety and depression, which led her deeper into destructive habits. But the food choices she made were never addressed as a way of possibly helping to make her life better. No one considered her gut health as a root cause of her low serotonin and imbalanced brain chemicals.

But your gut has an incredibly powerful impact on your brain. There is a direct physical connection between your brain and your gut by way of something called the Vagus nerve. It's one of the main nerves of your parasympathetic nervous system, and because your body wants to stay in that nice, relaxed parasympathetic nervous system state as much as it can, that nerve relays messages between your gut and your brain constantly. It provides a round-the-clock news-feed update about what's going on in the gut, so the brain can react accordingly, and vice versa.

This is why the gut is often called a "second brain." It's also why when you feel nervous, you experience "butterflies" in your stomach. Or why you feel like you have to run to the bathroom when you're anxious, stressed, or upset.

If you leave the surrounding nerves and take a deep dive directly into your gut to reach microscopic levels, you'll find a magnificent rainforest full of flora by way of bacteria. But don't be grossed out! These bacteria are beautiful for the incredible wonders they achieve for our bodies. Diversified colonies of bacteria populate in the gut, so they can support a highly functioning digestive system. Diversification is important! But there are "good microbes" and there are "bad microbes" that exist in our digestive tract, each thriving in their own way entirely depending on what we feed them. The goal is to feed the good microbes the feasts they need to prevent inflammation and to keep the gut cells healthy, so that the Vagus nerve can then report back to the brain that all is well.

We'll explore more about healthy diets for your gut later in this book, and you'll be amazed by what simple additions like probiotic and prebiotic foods can do for your energy, weight management, and mood. But this part of the book is all about listening to the signals your body is giving you, and your digestive system sure likes to talk!

Your gut has an incredibly powerful impact on your brain.

You can find and listen to your digestive system's signals in nearly every part of your body. It doesn't just talk by way of an upset stomach. It has the power to manifest signals in so many ways, so it's time to start paying attention to those signals.

For example, if your skin is consistently showing signs of irritation, your gut may not be healthy enough to remove toxins well, or it could be overreacting to foreign substances. If you notice a consistent dip in your mood after eating certain foods, especially those high in sugar and processed foods, it's because your gut becomes inflamed by these foods, and that link to your brain starts telling it to stop concentrating, feel irritated, or just get sleepy. And if you or your children get frequent colds or have low energy, your gut health is a great place to start looking for answers as to why.

Noticing what we eat and how it makes us feel, think, and act both directly after and into the next day is hugely important. When things are not working well in our gut, there will be clear signals. All it takes is focused attention to tune into this part of your body, and to what you consume. *Pinpoint what foods facilitate a clear mind, high energy, and a happy mood.* Also discern which foods do the opposite by creating brain fog, headaches, digestive upset, depleting energy, and souring your mood. These are real things that are a direct result of how we feed ourselves and our microbiome. These signals also reveal how well we are *actually absorbing the essential nutrients* from our food that our body needs to keep our systems and vital organs thriving.

To make these useful examinations, start by asking:

- How does my gut feel right now? Uncomfortable? Bloated? Painful? Sluggish? Overactive? Calm and satisfied? Productive and efficient?
- How is the sensation affecting my thoughts and mood? Am I anxious? Fatigued? Distracted? Unfocused? Irritated? Energized? Happy? Balanced? Content? Clear-minded?
- What did I eat today that could be making me feel this way?
- What are my consistent eating patterns and what do I physically experience because of them?

After years of careful practice with asking these questions, my own gut now almost immediately tells me when I've ingested something it's having problems with, in one way or another. I've determined my own diet based on these reactions, and in time I've learned to love everything my gut loves. *My favorite foods have become simple (and tasty!) foods that my body needs to consistently nourish and support my gut to work at its best. And because it absorbs all those whole food vitamins and powerfully rich nutrients, my body and my mind reward me with vibrant energy and focus.*

But it wasn't always that way. In the past, my digestive system did not work well. I was unaware of the foods that were aggravating it, and I had little knowledge of what my digestive tract thrived on, so I would often experience terrible bloating. It got to the point that I would unbutton my pants due to the pain – even if I was in public! It was exhausting and unpleasant, not to mention awkward…

Now, I've learned to pay attention to what my gut tells me after I've eaten certain foods. For example, chips and salsa are one of my favorite snacks. You'd never expect them to be the cause of any trouble. But if I fall into temptation and eat an entire bowl of chips, discomfort hits me in the middle of the night, preventing me from sleeping. In order not to toss and turn for the remainder of the night, I get up, lay on my bedroom floor, and start doing yoga body twists to relieve the discomfort so that I can return to bed and get back to sleep. Even though it works, who wants to do yoga in the middle of the night?! So, the better choice is to skip the chips and sleep like a baby. The best choice is always listening to what your gut really needs.

If your gut is happy, then the rest of your body will be energized and function well. That's why I like to call the foods that my body loves the most my "happy meals." In due time, you'll also learn what your own happy meals are, and more on how to achieve that will come later in this book. For now, just remember that your gut will signal to you when it's not healthy with symptoms in almost every system in your body. From there, you'll develop a habit of listening, investigating, and identifying your body's signals so you can make the changes you need to. Listening to your gut will empower you to confidently be the best advocate for your entire body.

The Respiratory System

You've likely heard the saying, "You are what you eat," and we've just learned there's a lot of truth to that. But I'd also add, "You are how you breathe!" This is because how you breathe not only determines how well you fuel your body with oxygen, but also the crispness of your mind, the strength of your muscles, and your immune response. Every system in the body relies on our oxygen. And listen to this: How you breathe can even affect the behavior of your central nervous system.

Your respiratory system usually functions without your input. You will keep on breathing whether you're thinking about it or not. But that doesn't necessarily mean you're breathing well. In fact, most people don't breathe in a way that allows the body to function optimally. So, when it comes to listening to your respiratory system in the sense of making it work better for your whole body on a lasting level, you need to address how you breathe and particularly take note how you breathe through the stressful moments when your sympathetic nervous system kicks into gear.

The best way to breathe first and foremost starts with great posture. Good posture helps the flow of air into the lungs and the removal of carbon dioxide out. Start by sitting up straight with your shoulders slightly back to help the lungs expand quickly and easily with every breath. You will experience an immediate improvement in how well oxygen reaches your bloodstream and your brain.

While many people focus on completely inhaling to improve their breathing, most people fail to realize that completely exhaling, and expelling as much carbon dioxide as possible during the process, is also important. So try hard to push all the air out of your lungs, as though you are blowing bubbles. Not only will your body reward you with instant energy, but you'll also notice how much more efficient you'll become at filling your lungs (Elliot Physical Therapy, 2017).

How you breathe can even affect the behavior of your central nervous system.

Intentional deep breathing is one of the best ways to calm yourself, even from the slightest bit of uneasiness, whether it happens in a conversation, work meeting, or grocery shopping with your children. For example, if I wake up at night and don't fall asleep within a few minutes, I feel myself getting concerned and uneasy. Focusing on my breathing and completing several quality breaths moves me back into a restful state and in no time, I'm back to sleep.

Now, when your sympathetic nervous system kicks into gear, if you can train your body to take deliberate, slow breaths through the stress, you can actually clamp down on that stress response like a mousetrap.

Ask yourself these questions during stressful moments, as well as in your normal, peaceful, parasympathetic nervous system state so that you can notice how you're breathing overall, and how you're breathing in stressful experiences:

- How much air is moving in and out of my lungs? A lot, or a little?
- How fast am I taking breaths?
- How does my chest feel? Tight or open? Fluttery or calm?
- How is my posture? Hunched or straight? What difference does opening my chest make to my breathing?
- How does my brain feel? Clear, foggy, or dizzy?
- What am I feeling emotionally as I'm breathing? Chaos, anxiety, fear, peace, calmness, concern, despair, contentment?

Answering these questions will clarify what you're experiencing, and what you need to do or change to support yourself in moving toward a more grounded parasympathetic state.

Sometimes, my fluttery chest comes on from changing up my morning coffee unknowingly to a stronger amount of caffeine. Or sometimes my tight chest or short breaths are a result of an unprocessed emotion trying to surface. So, noticing your signals and then identifying the potential stressor or catalyst behind them helps you understand how to calm yourself, support yourself, and make necessary changes. After a few buoyant breaths, or a brisk walk or jog where your lungs are filling and expanding well, check in with your emotions again. You will feel a difference!

The best way to breathe first and foremost starts with great posture.

Always remember, simply concentrating on the air coming in and out of your lungs can help your whole body relax, because oxygen has a restorative effect. Our bodies can't live without it, after all! Practicing deep breathing consistently will help develop your skill, and in time it will become a natural way of living for you. Just breathing effectively greatly enhances your wellbeing. Pretty amazing, isn't it?

The Musculoskeletal System

Your musculoskeletal system refers to the way your muscles, tendons, ligaments, and bones work together to support your body's movements. It's our framework, what holds us together and empowers us to live our lives with stability and force. Healthy muscles and bones aren't only vital to moving through life safely, but they give you the confidence to live life the way you want, and the controlled composure to make living that way a reality. If you're anything like me, you want to strengthen your musculoskeletal system, protect it, and maximize all the benefits it gives you!

A lot of confidence comes with innately knowing you can handle the physical challenges you experience in life, whether it be skiing down snowy slopes in Colorado, or just in the events of everyday life. For example, you might feel more confident taking your kids or grandchildren out to the park if you trust that your body can hop the fence to run after them when needed. Or you might get a boost of confident satisfaction when the helpful bagger at the grocery store offers to carry your heavy items to your car, but you graciously tell them you can carry them yourself.

Controlled composure means doing the actions in both those examples (and other scenarios you desire), without having to worry that your confidence about them might have gotten the better of you. Because in the moment, your muscles and bones perform the actions just as they needed to.

When it comes to supportive listening, your muscles and bones also supply important signals regarding your overall health. But they're not always as loud the way some of our other systems are. To learn how our musculoskeletal system is working with the rest of our systems, it takes some deliberate self-scanning, or what I like to call a "body scan."

You'll actually begin your body scan outside your own body. First, find a nice, quiet place to either sit or lie supine on the floor. Then, evaluate the week you've had so far. Has it been a balance of energizing activity and recharging your battery? Or has your week been an energy drain due to fatigued muscles from a lack of use and activity? Or, have you raced through every hour trying to reach your fitness goals, work goals, and meet your child's needs without realizing the tension building up within you as you go, go, go?

To start checking in on if and how that tension might exist, close your eyes and begin breathing. As you slow down your breath and your thoughts with intentional, rhythmic breaths, you'll feel relaxed. Now, focus first on the very crown of your head.

What are you physically feeling there? Once you've analyzed the area, slowly move your attention to your forehead, your face and jaw, your neck, and continue all the way down your body, right to your very toes. Stop to note and focus on any places that feel tight or painful in your muscles and bones. Take into account each side of your body as well. Where do you feel the differences in their strength and flexibility? Remember to let curiosity and compassion lead you. Just notice and accept right where you are without judgment. You're gathering valuable information to help you support your musculoskeletal system.

Note where you seem to hold your tension. Everyone carries it just a little differently, but some of the most common areas are in the neck, shoulders, back, and hips. Some people also tighten their jaw or clench their abdomen when they feel stressed. Personally, I was a jaw clencher for many years. I didn't realize that was the way my body manifested the stress and tension I hadn't released until I finally started exploring those areas more and tuned into what I really needed. Deep breathing, stretching all the muscles around the tight, tense areas, and rubbing dōTERRA Deep Blue® – a very restorative cream for aching muscles and sore joints – into my muscles became my bedtime routine. I haven't clenched my jaw in years, and my wellbeing is much better as a result.

Thinking back on your week, try to find the source of stress behind the tension, and then focus on relaxing your tight muscles by first implementing some of the slow, deep breathing you've already been doing that is so good for your body. Imagine yourself breathing new air and new life into those spaces, expanding them with a greater flow of oxygen. You may notice a difference in those tense areas of your body within just a few moments. Unprocessed, ongoing stress can stay locked in our tight muscles. A therapeutic muscle massage can soothe your muscles and identify stress. You may even experience some emotions surface as you begin to release the tension in these areas.

Once you start noticing the patterns of what causes stress and tension in your body and where you seem to carry most of it, then you can work to relieve that tension. Use this information in your body scans, and hear what your muscles, tendons, and joints are telling you throughout your day to create a targeted exercise and stretching routine, whether it includes joining a yoga class or doing it on your own. I recommend both! Your goal in creating your targeted exercise and stretching routine is to further reduce tension, loosen tight or painful muscles, improve balance, and build strength (more on that later).

Isn't this such an empowering way to listen to, treat, and better your body? All by drawing on your God-given intuition, focus, and willpower. This is the way we are designed to live, naturally in STRENGTH.

Know Your Numbers

Another valuable tool in helping you identify your body's signals is to find a physician that you trust and can partner with to care for your body. Combining their knowledge and experience with your own sources of information, your personal philosophy of health, and most importantly, your understanding of your own body, creates a powerful force for your best health as you collaborate.

I love partnering with a like-minded health-care physician to discuss my health goals and get a panel of specific lab work. Parts of your body, like your thyroid and your hormones, can communicate with you through some simple blood tests. Knowing the patterns of your hormone levels and thyroid levels is significant. It's important to follow and to understand your blood work results ("your numbers") and watch for trends. Blood-work findings will help you identify your body's signals for when you feel your best, and when something is imbalanced. Yes, there is so much to learn about our amazing bodies!

Find a physician that you trust and can partner with to care for your body.

A Natural Resource That Can Help

Sometimes you just can't beat some of the incredible pure, natural resources that are available these days to help you when you sense your body is signaling that it needs attention. One of my "go to" ways to help me reduce stress, or remedy a digestive system disturbance, or relieve musculoskeletal tightness and discomfort is by using essential oils. What are essential oils? They are natural extracts from the seeds, stems, roots, flowers, and other parts of plants.

CPTG Pure Therapeutic Tested Grade® essential oils, like dōTERRA oils, the brand I use, are the safest and purest. They are sourced from plants from around the world in order to provide the greatest benefits. But using essential oils safely is of utmost importance. Educating yourself and learning from someone who is experienced in using them is wise and necessary. I'm proud to say that I'm vastly experienced with and knowledgeable in essential oils, so I'm happy to help! Just reach out to me at my website: LyndaHebert.com/contact.

There are so many highly effective essential oils that can support your body's needs and your family's needs in every category of your health and wellbeing. I've experienced tremendous growth in supporting myself through using essential oils. In the *Action Table* at the end of this chapter, I list some of the essential oils to help you address some specific issues discussed in this chapter that your body may be signaling to you.

In Summary

Are you starting to notice just how much the systems in your body talk to you? Have you been able to recognize what they're trying to say? Learning this skill is not an overnight process, especially if you've been drowning out those voices for most of your life. A lot of us have been in the habit of ignoring our body's signals of stress, pain, discomfort, and poor health. And for you it may be because you don't even know what these signals are. So, it's naturally going to take some time to pinpoint exactly what's bothering you, and that's okay. As long as you keep listening to your body's dynamic processes with the intention of being as supportive to yourself as possible, you will get better and better at interpreting exactly what they're trying to say and what you need to do for them.

Check in with yourself daily. This can be as simple as pausing for a moment and asking:

- What am I physically experiencing right now?
- How's my gut doing and how is it speaking to me today?
- What does my breathing feel like?
- Are any of my muscles feeling tense?

This is all about noticing your own inner being signals and having no judgment about them as you do, as judgment will tempt you to be dishonest with yourself. This deep listening will open the door for you to support yourself at a cellular level, which can lead to better wellbeing and true health.

Welcome to your first "Action Points" chart! Going forward, at the very end of each chapter, you will find a concise chart explaining the specific Mindsets, Skillsets, and Toolsets relating to the topics we closely examined in the chapter. These charts contain all the important critical thinking and heart attitudes (Mindsets) of the chapter, the activities to do to practice supporting those mindsets (Skillsets), and the external tools I personally recommend for making achieving both of those much more attainable and sustainable (Toolsets).

After you've completed this book and are well into your STRENGTH journey, these Action Points will be great items to come back to in order to give yourself the refreshers you might need on all the things you've learned in this book!

Action Points: Supportive Listening: Sense Your Signals	
Mindset	• Develop and train your mind in deeper authentic listening to your body. Honor your body and express gratitude for how well it serves you. • Have an attitude of compassion and curiosity for and about yourself. • Don't place any judgement on yourself during this open, unhurried, and honest process.
Skillset	• Learn your body's sensations to find meaning, clarity, and patterns, as it relates to the particular body systems discussed in this chapter. Ask yourself these clarifying questions for each sensation and pattern you are recognizing: • What do I need and want more of, or less of? • What is giving me sustainable energy, and what is draining my energy? • What hurts my mental state, and what enhances my mood and focus? • Practice slow, deep breathing to achieve true, quality breathing.
	• Do body scans when trying to discover what your body is communicating

<table>
<tr><th colspan="2">Action Points:
Supportive Listening: Sense Your Signals</th></tr>
<tr><td>Toolset</td><td>
• Keep a record of these scans in your journal and reflect on them to notice patterns.
• Support yourself with essential oils to reduce stress and help shift out of irrational thinking patterns. Oils for focus and emotional balance as well when overwhelmed with worry and fear can include:
  o dōTERRA Peace® blend
  o Frankincense oil
  o dōTERRA Balance® blend
• Oils for digestive system disturbance:
  o dōTERRA DigestZen® blend
  o Peppermint oil
• Musculoskeletal tightness and discomfort
  o dōTERRA Deep Blue®
  o A therapeutic massage
• Partner with a like-minded licensed health-care provider to discuss your health goals and get a panel of specific lab work semi-annually. This helps you identify patterns with your hormone and thyroid levels and to track trends in your body's signals for when you feel your best and when something is imbalanced.
</td></tr>
</table>

You are so worth this! You can absolutely be your body's most supportive friend and healthcare provider if you develop the habit of listening to more clearly understand what your own body needs and *wants.* You can naturally restore and support yourself at a cellular level, which means addressing the root problem, not just fixing the surface symptoms. And when you're supported from within first, you'll reap a harvest of strength, beauty, and truth inside *and* outside yourself.

STRENGTH 4

Train Your Thought Patterns

Some people credit Abraham Lincoln with this famous quote: "Most folks are usually about as happy as they make their minds up to be." Whether he said it or not, I fully believe it.

Whatever you give your mindful attention to greatly expands in your experience. It's a powerful truth! If you dwell on your strengths, your blessings, your health goals, and all the people who love you, then you will attract even more blessings, even more love, and even more progress (Newberry, 2007). And inversely, if you dwell on your weaknesses, your fears, your obstacles, your poor health, and all the offenses you've experienced, then you'll draw more of that. Proverbs puts the same idea in another way that has always really resonated with me: "As a man thinks, so is he" (Proverbs 23:7 KJV).

To be healthy and well in life we must first think well. Our minds and the thoughts we think every day are unbelievably powerful. They can change the very course of our lives and the lives around us. Without a doubt, our consistent thoughts become our attitudes; our attitudes shape our day-to-day actions; our day-to-day actions form our lifestyle habits; our lifestyle habits become our character, the very essence of who we are. As John Locke says, "The actions of men are the best interpretations of their thoughts." This is why and how your mindset matters more than anything else when it comes to upgrading your life to one of thriving health.

These lifestyle habits shape and impact the quality of our very own wellbeing. Did you get that? Our thoughts determine our strength, vitality, and wellness! While challenges and hardships will always happen, our attitudes toward them can help ease the pain, bring about solutions, and all the while help us build resiliency in the process.

The first "T" in STRENGTH stands for "Train Your Thought Patterns." In this chapter, you will learn to think (and speak and act) in a manner that will bring about true health in every cell of your being. However, you must know: This chapter does *not* describe thinking the way *most* people think. Instead, this chapter is about thinking the way *few* people think, going against the flow so to speak. And if you want to be a part of this healthy "few", over time, hopefully we can turn it into the healthy "many".

So, first things first. We must start with ourselves. Training my own thoughts required discipline and consistent effort (and it continues to), because to be honest, I discovered that most of my disturbances, whether mental, spiritual, emotional, or physical originated from unproductive thoughts. And the thing is, when something is so naturally powerful in that way, learning how to use that power in the most effectively positive way takes some serious attention, training, and focus. I like how Ken Blanchard, the Co-author of the *One-Minute*

Manager, says it, "If you want to go places you've never been before – you have to think in ways you've never thought before."

So, allow this chapter to expand your mind, stretch your comfort zone, and gently move you away from the hazards that limit your true wellbeing.

Capture Your Thoughts

Without a doubt, the first step in training your thoughts is to become aware of and to notice your thoughts. In other words, "capture" your thoughts.

We have random thoughts all day, and we tend to repeat the same thoughts day after day. But we actually do *not* have to be subject to our own thoughts. When you are thinking thoughts such as *it's too late for me to change,* and *I don't believe I can change,* these are the kinds of thoughts that you want to capture (and replace).

Capturing your thoughts can begin with asking yourself some questions. This is not only a powerful way to determine what your thoughts are, but also an effective way to shape your thoughts. When in the process of asking and answering these questions, honestly acknowledge and accept your thoughts right where you are:

- What is the first thing I think about when I wake up in the morning? This is something you will naturally notice in time. How does that thought make me feel? What occupies my thoughts as I'm getting ready for my day? These thoughts set our mood and attitude for the day.

- As I encounter more emotions in a situation, what am I telling myself when in the midst of it? For example:
    - When I'm stressed about juggling all my responsibilities at work, the diverse needs of my young children, or the rising prices of everything around me.
    - When I'm feeling frustrated about my weight and not having enough time to consistently exercise.
    - When I'm upset about my mistakes or weaknesses that hurt me and others (or at least, I think they do).
- What am I thinking about before falling asleep at night? These thoughts can greatly affect our quality of sleep.

Once you've started readily recognizing what your most prevalent thoughts are, it's important to identify where these thoughts come from. What has fed this diet? In other words, understanding why you're thinking a certain way, or why you're telling yourself certain things. Every decision you make is either directly or indirectly impacted by your thought diet, so you need to understand it. As you evaluate what you're feeding your mind, consider these questions:

- What people in my life contribute to the way I think and feel?

- What events in my life cause these thoughts and feelings?
- What TV shows, news broadcasts, online reading, social media, movies, and books do I engage in regularly that contribute to my habits of thinking?

The things that we've consistently *allowed,* passively or intentionally, to make way into our hearts and minds sway our beliefs, feelings, values, expectations, and actions to a much greater degree than many of us are probably comfortable acknowledging. And when you decide to courageously tune in to yourself, listen to your mental chatter, and understand what is truly behind any repeated unhealthy thought (i.e., self-defeating, fearful, or untrue), which we all struggle with at times, you will be on your way to creating and sustaining a healthy, life-giving mindset.

Why Choose Our Thoughts?

Does the phrase "just do it" sound familiar? Regardless of if it does or doesn't, the reality is, we can't just "do" anything without thinking first. Every decision we make and action we take stems from thinking about it first, even if it's a subconscious one. We're designed that way. So, if our thoughts are what truly drive us, why not choose them and shape them to become the best version of ourselves possible?

You see, we tell ourselves certain truths and untruths in our thoughts, and they go on to affect the way we live. For example, I've discovered a repetitive thought that constantly urges me to work harder, move faster, and take shortcuts. Precisely, my thought that *"there isn't enough time"*, or *"I don't have enough time"* constantly drives me when I allow it to. This twisted thought produces stress and anxiety within me. But I don't really believe this thought is accurate, so I continue to work at investigating it and replacing it with a more truthful one. I'm working at shifting that thought to: *"I'm learning to prioritize what I do each day I'm given and invest my time in what I value most."* Again, you want *your* thoughts to be guided by *your* true core beliefs. But if you're like me, often they are not. And that's what needs to change.

Thankfully, by the way God designed us, we have the freedom to intentionally *choose* our thoughts with a plan and a disciplined method of regulating what we dwell on. And that plan and method we habitually choose day after day will create a life of truthful, purposeful, healthful living. But before we talk about that plan and method, there are some important things to understand about how our brain responds to our thoughts.

The Science Behind Training Our Thought Patterns

Our minds are hardwired to keep us safe. They're going to do what they feel they need to do to that end, and often that involves prompting us to stick with what is normal or with what's *familiar* to us. Think about how you feel when you explore something like a new walking trail; you're not sure where it's taking you or what you might encounter. It's new and different, and until you walk that same trail over and over, you might not feel safe and free on it. That's because our mind thinks what is familiar *is* what is safe. And because what is familiar *feels* safe, our brain thinks that what we have repeatedly done *is* safe. And so, it prompts us to continue doing more of the same.

So, we need to help our brain get more comfortable with what is *unfamiliar* to us. And this requires faith. Establishing new thoughts actually feels abnormal and unnatural (I feel this way anytime I replace old thoughts with new ones), and it doesn't happen overnight. You may need to let go of some thoughts that previously brought you comfort. Thoughts that are counterproductive need to be discarded. We need to learn to step out of our self-made comfort zone so we can grow stronger and healthier. And the only way to do that is to slowly stretch the lines of our comfort zone and start taking new steps beyond those familiar paths we unknowingly created. Yes, it's challenging. But replacing lies with truth (by establishing a new way of thinking) brings indescribable life-giving freedom!

We can reshape our neural pathways, meaning we can change the way our brain thinks and functions. Back when my sister was having persistent mental health issues, my family was told that the chemicals produced by her brain (and all human brains) were a fixed, undynamic entity, and as such, the imbalances in her brain were permanent and unchangeable. They also said the way our brain circuitry works, including our nerve pathways, is constant and immutable. But today, we realize just how untrue that is. So much science and research now show that our brains are malleable.

This concept is called "neuroplasticity," and it explains how our thoughts are moldable. By definition, neuroplasticity is "the ability of the brain to form and recognize synaptic connections, especially in response to learning or experience" (Oxford Languages). Synaptic connections are the parts of our brains that connect the whole organ together, where information about how to think and function is passed along, and there are millions of them in a single brain. Through neuroplasticity, the brain can be rewired to function in some way that differs from how it previously functioned. That means we can be our own microsurgeons as we make choices that will change the very circuits in our brains!

Through this "self-brain surgery," we can rewire our brains by actively choosing to think differently; to literally change our minds. And the more we reinforce a new way of thinking, the more those new synaptic connections shift and grow, resulting in changes in our thoughts, emotions, and actions.

We can reshape our neural pathways, meaning we can change the way our brain thinks and functions.

Neuroscientists have determined that every thought sends electrical and chemical signals throughout your brain, ultimately affecting each cell in your body. Thoughts can influence your sleep, your digestion, your pulse, the chemical makeup of your blood, and all other bodily bodily functions

(Newberry, 2007). When our thought patterns are truly healthy, we have more energy, joy, and high-quality systemic functioning within our cells.

What You Say to Yourself Matters

In the previous chapter, we discussed how vitally important it is to listen to yourself. But it's also equally important to know how to *talk* to yourself.

What do you believe about yourself? The way you talk about yourself to yourself matters – a lot! "The highest form of individual responsibility is responsibility for our thought life; all mental work is delayed, and all upward progress is deferred until this is acknowledged" (Newberry, 2007). Decide first and foremost your standard for how you repeatedly talk to yourself every day and allow that same philosophy to carry into all your conversations with others.

There are lies circulating all around us that are masqueraded as truth, about what will make us (and our children) happy, healthy, successful, or valuable. We need to decide for ourselves what unchanging beliefs we hold onto, so that we can recognize those traps of thinking that eventually bring distress and diseased cells.

Think This, Not That

Once you do know those beliefs and standards, it's time to replace those unhealthy, non-productive thoughts with ones that are life-giving, useful, and effective for bringing about the changes you want to see in your life. This is an ongoing daily habit. Think about *what you want,* not what you *don't* want. By doing so, you actively reinforce your mind to think something else, thereby taking advantage of neuroplasticity and rewiring your brain to have better thoughts. When those new synapses are built, you eventually won't have to work so deliberately to do so. Choice by choice, day by day, it will become an automatic habit.

Some examples of how to replace your current mental diet with a healthier diet may include:

- Replacing "It's too late for me to change" with "It's never too late to change" and "I know I can!"
- Replacing "Yesterday was a disaster so today is going to be worse," with "Yesterday was a valuable learning experience that will make today much more productive."
- Replacing "I'm so frustrated with my aching back and tight muscles," with "I'm so grateful for all the things that work well in my body, and I know I have the potential to improve."
- Cultivate compassionate thoughts, not harsh ones.
- Think successful thoughts, not failing thoughts.
- Think about the joy of eating tasty, healthy foods, not the short-term gratification of eating junk food.
- Think about how energized you'll feel when you're done with your 30-minute run or power walk, not about how you're too tired to exercise.

- Think about the calm spirit and clear wisdom you'll experience for days, instead of the sense of unproductivity you initially feel as you choose to spend most of your day resting and reflecting quietly.
- Think about pushing the "pause" button and the calmness that will come, instead of your overwhelming urge to "react."

Establish boundaries for yourself, as it relates to what triggers unhealthy thoughts. Yes, I know from experience, when we neglect to establish boundaries to protect ourselves, or don't honor them, we open the door for unproductive thoughts. I've learned through experience, when I don't take time away to shut down my mind (for about 30 minutes each day), giving myself the opportunity to recharge and regain perspective, my mind becomes weak. And I'm more prone to reactive or unproductive thoughts. Also, too much social media can release some unsettling anxiety within me, either because I'm wasting my time or it's just not productive. So, I've learned to be aware of how I navigate social media, ensuring I do it in a way that benefits my mind.

Set your disciplines that support your thought-life goals and follow them, because the more you build your disciplines to create a positive thought life, the stronger you'll get.

It's vital that we guard our minds because our thoughts affect everything about us.

Everyone's new mental diet will look a little different based on what their current diet consists of, where their thoughts have been coming from, and what they want to achieve in life. But that's the incredible thing about how our minds work: *You* are in complete control. *You* choose and shape your thoughts. No one else can do that or has the power to choose your thoughts for you. It is God-given!

Building a Disciplined Mental Diet

Practice and repetition are key when it comes to changing our mental diet, because that's the way a new habit is formed. Remember, consistent repetition brings about incremental changes that eventually become an automatic habit, which eventually internalizes as part of our identity. Training your thoughts is no different. And that's what living in STRENGTH is all about!

The first step is to guard your mind actively and offensively regarding the thoughts you allow in. People guard their homes, cars, and belongings from outside and threatening intrusions because of their value to them. For example, you wouldn't leave your front door open or your car keys in your ignition for any length of time – that would be inviting trouble in. But how even more valuable is your mind!

It's vital that we guard our minds because our thoughts affect everything about us. In other words, protect what enters your "mental workshop," where you have those private, top-secret conversations with yourself. What seeps into our minds shows up in those inward conversations, and those conversations make a huge impact on our actions, habits, and wellbeing. Our minds need protection against inflammatory triggers and unwanted scripts sneaking in.

The next step is to intentionally expose yourself to all the best influences you know every day, until it's an automatic habit. Some examples of how to do this can include:

- Whatever strengthens and fortifies your mind the most, dwell on and marinate in that daily, as it will bring you wholeness and health (for me, it's life-giving truth and wisdom of the Scriptures).
- Watching TV shows, news broadcasts, online videos, social media, and movies that contribute to healthy habits of thinking.
- Listening to uplifting or educational Podcasts and radio stations (changing it up stimulates a growth mindset).
- Listening to music that promotes the mindset you want.
- Reading books that enrich your mind and strengthen your entire being.
- Making time to connect with and talk to someone every day who you know will motivate you, encourage you, and tell you the truth.
- Scheduling classes, seminars, and retreats that help you improve your focus and renew your thought life.

Again, you will have a specific mental diet that makes *you* uniquely healthy. We are diverse in our backgrounds and experiences, so all of our diets will look a little different. The important thing is to be honest (and over time you will know if you are), about the mental diet that undoubtedly makes you the best version of yourself.

Action Points: Train Your Thought Patterns	
Mindset	• Cultivate the mindset that aligns with your core values and beliefs. • Take seriously what you say to yourself, and how you say it, as this matters greatly to your wellbeing. • Understand that achieving a state of a productive and healthy "mind diet" takes practice.
Skillset	• Recognize your dominant thoughts. • Understand where those thoughts have come from. • Deliberately replace unhealthy thoughts with healthier, more productive thoughts. • Learn how to guard and protect your mind. • Continue surrounding yourself with the people, places, ideas, principles and truths from the books, messages, broadcasts, and other inputs that provide highly nourishing thought-food for your mental diet.

Action Points: ***Train Your Thought Patterns***	

Toolset	• Write about your thoughts and mental diet in your journal.
	• Refer to your vision board to find healthy thoughts to replace old ones.
	• Breathing, movement, and meditation can help you gain calm clarity.
	• Prayer can help you achieve clarity, inspiration, and motivation.
	• Books that can fuel an excellent mental diet, such as:
	  ○ The Bible (ESV Version)
	  ○ *Atomic Habits* by James Clear
	  ○ *Switch On Your Brain* by Dr. Caroline Leaf
	  ○ *The 4:8 Principle* by Tommy Newberry
	  ○ *Anatomy of the Soul* by Dr. Curtis Thompson
	  ○ *Strengthsfinder* by Don Clifton, from the Gallup Strengths Assessment
	  ○ *Own your Own Mind* by Andrew Carnegie.
	• Essential oils such as frankincense, sandalwood, lemon, and peppermint in particular help with focus and clarity.

Our amazing human mind is where we create, organize, and build our unique thoughts, and where we crystallize which thoughts empower us to be holistically healthy and fueled by our greatest aspirations and passions. This ultimately brings great value to everyone around you, the next generation, and possibly to the entire world. Your thoughts and my thoughts matter, so let's choose them, develop them, and build them carefully!

Replacing lies with truth (by establishing a new way of thinking) brings indescribable life-giving freedom.

---

5 ST(R)ENGTH

Rest and Rejuvenate

I have a question I would love to ask: When was the last time you felt deeply rested in body, mind, and spirit?

For me, earlier in life, I would have had trouble answering that question because I lacked any insight into the value of true rest. And maybe this is where you are today; not clear about how to effectively rest, and not convinced rest is even necessary, except for when you're completely exhausted. Like I once believed, you may be too busy to stop and take time to fill your rapidly emptying tank. And before you know it, you find yourself running on fumes and wondering how you got there.

In our fast paced, always-on culture, it's easy for people to convince themselves that rest isn't important, and often believe that doing *something* is more productive than, well, doing nothing. And it's easy to conclude that pushing through all our activities somehow makes us tougher. However, science has been gathering steam in proving what should have been intuitive all along: rest is central to our health and performance (Oura, 2023).

You're about to discover the hidden gem of true rest. That's why I'm beaming with pleasure over sharing this chapter with you! I personally discovered, through having little choice but to rest, the richly restorative, life enhancing, and growth-producing benefits that rest brings. It's truly amazing! Most people don't fully understand or appreciate the enormous benefits of restoration and renewal that rest produces. But just like me, by the time you're done with this chapter, you'll love intentionally scheduling rest into your days, and you'll also enjoy getting to discover and appreciate what true rest looks like for you. Because contrary to popular belief, rest does not just refer to sleeping. There are *so* many ways to renew, restore, and rejuvenate your mind, body, and soul, and we're going to discover what they are and how they can all be useful to living in STRENGTH.

You'll see that once you *give yourself permission to rest* (yes, this is what actually holds many of us back from seeking the rest we need), the discovery of experiencing renewing rest within you can begin. Your sense of awe and wonder will be reawakened, and your creative juices will flow. And then, without a doubt, you will deeply value practicing your habit of rest!

The Impact of Rest on Your Health

While quality sleep is critical to feeling whole, rest is so much more than your nightly hours of sleep. Rest involves your whole being, not just your body. With complete and regular rest, you will restore your health, enhance your performance, and achieve an amazing sense of wellness (AdventHealth, 2021). Rest is vital for better mental health, increased concentration and memory, a healthier immune system, reduced stress, and even better metabolism (Integris Health, 2021).

The Science of Rest

Our bodies are not made to "do it all" all the time. That's not to say we don't have it in us to do big things in our lives, because we absolutely do! It just means that we need an ebb and flow. We need time to relax because our body's biology requires it of us. And we can find evidence of that fact by understanding something called our circadian rhythms.

The National Institute of Health defines circadian rhythms as "physical, mental, and behavioral changes that follow a 24-hour cycle. These natural processes respond primarily to light and dark and affect most living things, including animals, plants, and microbes" (NIH, 2023).

Our circadian rhythms are part of our larger biological clocks, which control and regulate many of the functions of our bodies. They time things like hormone releases, body temperature, and even our eating habits and digestion. For women, the release of estrogen in our bodies is extremely reliant on circadian rhythms. But where most people notice and unintentionally manipulate their circadian rhythms is in their sleep patterns.

When the optic nerves in our eyes receive information via the light outside, and that light gets dimmer (meaning day is turning to night), our body releases melatonin to make us tired and prepare us to sleep through the night. If we mess with that rhythm, such as by forcibly staying awake when we're tired, or sitting in front of a bright, blue-light screen right before bed, it can really mess up our sleep!

Though nighttime sleep is a major element of circadian rhythms, there are many more ways to connect to those rhythms and utilize them all throughout the day in order to give yourself the right amount of energy to get things done, but without overwhelming yourself. If you can understand and use daily rhythms of rest effectively, you can plan time for your hormones to calm down so you can reconnect to your intuition and reap the benefits of your body resting and repairing itself.

We need to find a way to make the most of these restful, reparative moments so that our bodies are working optimally, and our mind and spirit are thriving. Thankfully, there are so many great ways to do just that, and we will explore those soon!

What Happens When Rest Is Not a Priority

You might already know the importance of rest, but it's important to understand specifically the impact a lack of rest can have on your health.

When your body's core needs of rest and repair are not met, it can't help but underperform mentally and physically, and will increasingly react in undesirable ways. This often shows up in our work and in our relationships. Your ability to solve problems, be creative, and use good thinking declines as your crucial decision-making center, the prefrontal cortex, reduces activity. Meanwhile, your brain's emotional center, the amygdala, increases activity. That means you're more likely to overreact to social situations, such as a fight with your spouse (Oura, 2023). If you're a mother, you may have even seen this occur in your overtired children when they fight with their siblings.

Remember: Health is a process, not a singular event.

Also, when our bodies feel depleted by overworking and under resting, we are more prone to inflammation in our gut, which weakens our immune system and makes us more vulnerable to viruses and illness. In addition, we become more prone to injuries such as tripping, as our sense of balance and muscle strength reduces.

The necessary sense of balance that sets you up to be capable, sturdy, focused, and resilient physically, mentally, and spiritually, comes from meeting your needs with high quality prioritized habits – like the ones we're learning about on our road to STRENGTH.

And one of those most important habits is rest.

The body needs time to repair itself but cannot do so unless it's in a parasympathetic state (which you're already familiar with!). The body needs times of calmness and relaxation to repair its tissues and organs, which in turn repairs all its functions.

Remember: Health is a process, not a singular event. We are in constant need of purification to reach that goal, and the only way there is to allow our bodies the *time and rest* they need.

The Rhythms of Rest

If we take a close look at our circadian rhythms, we can see just how important rhythm is to our wellbeing. This is why I like to recommend building rhythms into your rest as well. Your body will tell you when it needs to rest, but you can build your own rhythm in before it even reaches that point and make the most of it!

For some of us, this requires more discipline than others. It's important to understand yourself and see your patterns. For example, high achievers can find it demotivating to rest. For example, if you take the StrengthsFinder Test and "Achiever" is one of your top-five strengths, that means you get a lot of satisfaction, drive, and motivation from accomplishing your goals and tasks. However, this also means that because you are a high achiever, someone like you *especially* needs time to refill your cup. You *need* rest to recharge yourself and renew that excitement and motivation for your next task or goal to accomplish. It's so important to refresh yourself and refuel your tank. Rest is extremely important for you!

Think about how you want to rest on a daily, weekly, monthly, quarterly, and yearly basis. Resting every day is critical, but it's so important to take breaks from your regular routine too. Weekly changeups of your rest routine, monthly getaways or outings, and yearly vacations are all important rhythms to build into your rest schedule.

Note a study-based *New York Times* article titled "Relax! You'll be More Productive!" The writer states that studies on rest have found "[m]ore time away from the office and longer, more frequent vacations boost productivity, job performance and, of course, health" (Schwartz, 2013).

These findings, along with other studies, continue to accentuate the benefits of regular rest and rejuvenation for your job performance, whether in your career in the workplace or your job at home caring for your family.

The most important aspect of rest is being intentional with it, so plan it and schedule it to make it a habit. Begin with daily rhythms that promote a peaceful start to your day. Plan the morning rhythm and evening rest routine. That could mean starting your day listening to inspiring music, invigorating exercise, or doing some meditation on what fuels your soul. This could be an all-in-one package, as it is for me.

An evening rest routine could include fifteen minutes of stretching followed by an Epsom salt bath with lavender oil (again, as I like to do). This sets you up for a refreshing night's sleep and a bountiful start to the following day.

Next, think about your weekly rhythms of rest, or the slightly larger restful activity you will do once per week. Maybe it's going out to the beach to watch the tide roll in. Maybe it's getting a soothing massage, a pedicure, curling up in a corner of a coffee shop to read or to journal some fresh ideas and thoughts. Maybe it's having a date night with your spouse or a catch-up conversation with a close friend.

Whatever it is, make it something you find so utterly restorative that you look forward to it every single week.

Monthly rest could involve a quick trip out of a town away from your normal regular routine, as this naturally refreshes your spirit and renews perspectives.

Your quarterly rest might be a slightly longer trip, getting away with your spouse or family for some fun and relaxation.

And your yearly rest might be several different weeklong vacations (or longer) absorbed in doing what you love and the people you love to be with. These trips are needed to deeply restore and replenish you, and what they consist of will change depending on the season you've just experienced. They might involve deep reflection in a beautiful setting, or a vacation of playing and adventuring with family or friends by doing your favorite activities in spectacular surroundings.

Thankfully, rest creates the perfect natural environment for our bodies to restore, replenish, repair, and rejuvenate all parts of ourselves so that we're ready to continue embracing our lives with a full cup brimming with energy and joy!

All the Wonderful Ways to Rest

As mentioned, there are so many productive ways to rest your body other than sleep. In fact, in this section, I'm not going to talk about sleep at all! We'll save that for a little later and instead focus on some of my absolute favorite additional ways to seek out the renewing rest your body needs daily and throughout your seasons of life. Because in some seasons, such as having a baby, caring for an infant, battling an illness, or experiencing some kind of trauma, it will be even more imperative to support yourself with constant rest and restorative practices.

In no particular order, below are some of my absolute favorite ways to rest throughout daily life and as seasons change. They can be extremely beneficial to anyone to try and experiment with. It's all about finding the kind of rest that's most restorative for you.

Reflection

Focused periods of time meant for intense thinking might sound like a lot of work, but they can in fact be restful in the same way that daydreaming can. That's because in order to enter this state of focusing the mind, we must slow our bodies down, be still, and still the world around us. This does wonders for our mental health and wellbeing.

Ask yourself what makes you come alive in your spirit. Is it nature? Listening to classical music? Praying? Creating? Adventure? Being with people you love? Meditating on your core beliefs? Notice what calms you, refreshes you and rejuvenates you like nothing else. Add these findings into your rhythms of rest.

Journaling is an excellent way to practice reflection. Putting your fragmented thoughts, feelings, and concerns into words on paper can give you the perspective you need.

Another way to reflect is to shift into a perspective of gratitude. This means searching and scanning your mind for simple everyday things you are grateful for. Believe me, I have those days when I do not feel like being thankful for anything. But even on those days, when I take time to deliberately contemplate all the things around me that I am grateful for, miraculously, my feelings of gratitude about everything become natural. Develop the habit of looking for and expressing gratitude. It's huge for your overall mental health and integrated wellness.

Yet another way you might choose to reflect is while being alone by yourself, with no agenda except to listen to your mind, heart, and spirit. This gives you the space you need to discover what truly renews and restores you. Notice the beauty around you if you're at the beach or in the mountains. In all your most potentially restorative places, create beauty. You'll love how this soothes and relaxes you. Your bedroom, your office, your kitchen, and the area you relax in – fill them with what speaks beauty to your mind and soul. Even your car can be a place of reflection – it often is for me.

Movement

Again, moving might seem like a strange way to rest, but it's true! If the movement you choose isn't particularly rigorous or physically exhausting (though that kind of movement certainly has an important place on the path to STRENGTH), it can put your mind and body into a peaceful, restful state that can be absolutely rejuvenating.

Yoga is perhaps one of the best examples of powerfully restorative movement. We'll talk more extensively about yoga and how it's beneficial later in this book, but when it comes to renewing and replenishing our minds and bodies, there are specific restful yoga movements and flows that are meant to nourish the parasympathetic nervous system and allow the body repair naturally. They help to unwind tension in your vital organs, nourish your adrenal glands, and some poses even help regulate hormones. This movement can also cultivate a still mind, which is essential for rest.

You can also find rest through movement in other ways, such as heading outdoors to be in nature. One of my absolute favorite ways to achieve rest through movement is to go for a walk outside. When I'm out in the open air, where I can feel and hear the windy breeze around me and gaze up into the bright blue sky, I notice the shifts that take place within me. My mind becomes clearer, my muscles feel more relaxed, and my breathing slows down. All of this contributes to mental clarity, healthier cellular functioning, and achieving a heart that's at peace.

Finally, one of the most calming ways to utilize movement to achieve rest is through deep breathing. Yes, breathing can also be considered active and deliberate movement of your body that can counteract stress responses by summoning your parasympathetic nervous system to bring your body to a relaxing state and restore equilibrium. When you take in more oxygen, your heart rate slows, and your mind calms down, allowing your body and spirit to replenish themselves.

Meditation

There is an *incredible* amount of science behind the ways that meditation can bring us into a restful state and actively renew so many parts of our bodies. Elizabeth Blackburn, a Nobel baccalaureate and biochemist at the University of California San Francisco, along with additional scientist and psychiatrist colleagues, have conducted research that has linked meditation to reducing inflammatory activity, increasing positive antiviral response, improving function of specific strands of immune cells, and achieving higher antibody production (Blackburn et al., 2009).

Yet, many people misunderstand or misjudge what meditation is and can be. It simply includes stillness, silence, space, and surrender. It's meant first and foremost to be a mind-body-soul practice that is richly renewing and restorative to all parts of our being. We just need to take the mysticism out of meditation.

Yes, it's been around a long time, and many of us have in fact been meditating without realizing it because simply being still and being fully present in the moment, as you focus on your life-giving breath, can deeply restore you. All the while, dwelling on one of your deepest core beliefs, such as "I am deeply known and loved," and letting all other thoughts pass by you, is a powerful form of meditation.

Meditation has become a huge component of rest for me. Several days a week, I have a planned period of meditation. However, I have also adopted a way of meditating into my lifestyle as I'm soaking in quiet moments, absorbing the beauty of what my senses are experiencing, stretching my body while mindfully breathing, or visualizing my future.

Adopting a routine of meditation into your life takes practice.

Prayer

Prayer and meditation have similarities because they both involve the moment when our soul feels integrated with our entire being. This can be an extremely restorative state to reach.

For me, praying, connecting with God, and specifically telling him (although he already knows) all my needs, desires, hopes, and fears, and placing my trust in his power, is replenishing. Exercising my faith in that way completely renews me.

I like to recommend prayer to rest because I know that when I over-strive (as I often do) and eventually come face-to-face with a lack of productivity as a result, reaching peace about that situation can be difficult. But spending this special time in quiet solitude and connecting with God, who made me and wants me to see what He sees, does wonders for my mind, body, and soul. Jesus so gently reminds us, "*Come to me all who are weary and heavy laden, and I will give you rest.*" This restores my very essence and gives my heart true peace.

Natural Tools and Resources

There is also an abundance of extraordinary, natural resources and tools accessible today that are invaluable in promoting rest and relaxation.

When it comes to releasing the tension that builds up in my body because of the stresses I'm experiencing in life, I love taking Epsom salt baths. A pure Epsom salt bath will renew you like nothing else! Epsom salt is also known as bath salt and is made of magnesium sulfate. It's entirely different from regular table salt, and its helpful minerals can be absorbed. Low magnesium levels have been shown to negatively affect sleep quality and stress (Elliot, 2023), so adding more of it to your life can be truly restful. Just add one or two cups of Epsom salt to a warm bath and soak in it for as long as you can – even if it's only ten minutes. This is a huge way to support and rest your muscles and your mind.

One of my favorite ways to support all parts of myself is by using essential oils (discussed back in Chapter 3). There are many highly effective essential oils that can aid with rest and relaxation. The essential oils I predominately use are lavender oil, dōTERRA Serenity® blend, and dōTERRA Peace® blend.

I also enjoy getting deep tissue massages and find them even more effective with the help of a restorative cream called dōTERRA Deep Blue®. When you rub it into your aching muscles, sore joints, or inflammatory areas of your body, you'll be amazed by the release of tension in those places and the relief of your aching pain. Deep Blue® has been life-changing for me in the way it reduces the tension, tightness, and inflammation in my muscles, therefore reducing my discomfort dramatically! And when our discomfort is reduced, more restful healing can take place.

Whichever method of rest you decide to give a try, notice how your body responds to each one. Tune in to what you experience both in the moment and beyond, and what happens inwardly for you on every level. Rest is unique for everyone. Discover your favorite "rest recipes," what brings you mental relaxation and what calms your body physically, and then do more of it. Schedule it into your life, and eventually it will become automatic!

So Where Does Sleep Fit In?

I promised we would talk about sleep, and I haven't forgotten! While it's true that there are so many useful ways to rest, the sleep you get is, of course, the most effective and important way to truly rest and renew your body so it can keep helping you do everything you love in life.

It's first important to understand the science of how your body works while you're sleeping. You might notice that if you don't sleep well at night, the next day you may feel depleted and achy. That's because your body didn't have the restful time it needed to restore all your physical and mental processes.

Consistent, quality sleep is one of the best ways to keep your body thriving. During nighttime sleep, a part of your circadian rhythm enacts that tells your body to do all the major cleaning and maintenance it needs to stay healthy. Your truest and deepest healing takes place during this time: Your wounds are worked on, your brain reorganizes the events and the memories from the day before, your digestive system resets itself. These are just a few examples of the work that your body is doing while you're sleeping – and it can only do at its highest possible level specifically *when* your body is sleeping. It's the best medicine of all!

It's imperative that we guard our nightly sleep as the sacred thing that it is. And we can do that by learning how to treat our bodies to prepare us for good, consistent sleep. Your bedtime routine is so important here. Creating consistent, helpful actions you take before going to bed each night will help you fall asleep more easily and stay asleep through the night so you can feel refreshed the next day.

Consistent, quality sleep is one of the best ways to keep your body thriving.

You've already been given an array of restful tools to try as part of your new bedtime routine. Any of the activities detailed as wonderful ways to rest are great for easing your body and mind into a restful state that understands it's almost time for bed. Your circadian rhythm will already get things started for you by releasing melatonin when the sun goes down, and you can help it by further removing yourself from light, such as TVs, computers, and phone screens at least one hour before bed. Instead, use that hour to do something you've discovered as truly restful, such as yoga, journaling, reading, prayer … you name it!

Find the most effective wind-down method for you, and then stick to it. You'll be amazed by how quickly you'll lull your body into sleep, and how peaceful that sleep will be. Then, staunchly guard that routine. Besides your newborn baby's needs or the occasional needs of your children, fiercely protect your nightly sleep so you can get the restoration mind, body, and soul all need. Remember: With full and consistent rest, you will improve your performance, restore your health, and experience an amazing feeling of wellness.

Action Points: Rest and Rejuvenate	
Mindset	• Develop a love for rest by embracing it fully and understanding its benefits. • Also understand that rest comes in many forms—not just sleep—and many of them are important to implement into your daily life. • Set boundaries for your rest, then guard and protect them closely.
Skillset	• There are so many unique ways to achieve rest (see Toolset below), and it's about experimenting with them until you find the types that are most renewing for you. • Once you've discovered your best rest methods, build them into the rhythms of your life on a daily, weekly, monthly, quarterly, and yearly basis. • Develop a truly restful bedtime routine and then stick to it consistently so that you can experience the most rejuvenating sleep possible and give your body what it needs to fuel you through the next day.

Action Points: Rest and Rejuvenate	
Toolset	• A journal, books, or the Bible can all provide meaningful rest. • Music • Deep breathing • Movement (like walks and yoga) • Meditation • Prayer • Epsom salt baths • Essential oils such as dōTERRA lavender oil, Serenity® blend, and Peace® blend. • dōTERRA Deep Blue® cream • A sleep tracker like an Oura, which measures the amount of REM sleep, deep sleep, and overall amount of sleep you're getting at night. It also measures your heart rate patterns correlating it to your rest and recovery each day.

Ahhh! Isn't this an amazing way to live? Rest is so peaceful and invigorating, it's a wonder to me that more people don't take advantage of it! Don't be afraid of rest – it's going to give you everything you need to succeed on this journey to STRENGTH (and more!).

Listen to the signals your mind and body are giving you, consider your needs carefully, find the restful activities that work best for you, and you will be able to give yourself the very best rest that your amazing body needs to help you live each day as your best day.

6 STRENGTH

Exercise and Move

Would you be surprised if I told you there was something you could do that only takes a few minutes to accomplish each day, but has the potential to significantly reduce your risk of things like cancer, stroke, type 2 diabetes, depression, anxiety, and if you're a woman, it can even help protect you from osteoporosis?

You might be surprised that something that takes so little time could have so much impact, but would you still be surprised if I told you that thing was … exercise? Probably not! And that's because most people know that exercise is extremely beneficial to their health.

But what they don't know is that even doing just a little bit of it on a *consistent* schedule can go a long way. So instead, many people think of working out as an exhaustive chore that batters their body in the name of "no pain, no gain." But the reality is, exercise doesn't need to be painful or even exhausting to be effective. Even simple exercises can keep your heart strong, build the muscles that make everything work, and enhance the flexibility and agility that goes with that.

Too much pain is *not* gain, so you don't need to think of exercise as a grueling or unpleasant part of your daily routine.

Instead, achieving the right dose of exercise and effort will be a new key to success, and this chapter is all about demonstrating just how true that is when navigating your road to STRENGTH.

What Happens When We Exercise

Our bodies love movement! That's because more movement requires more oxygen to be delivered to your cells, so when you move, you get more delicious oxygen coursing through your body. Oxygen is our body system's lifeline, so with more of it, your body becomes happier through and through. That's one of the reasons why you feel so elated during and after taking part in exercise, whether it's walking, swimming, dancing, or anything in between.

Of course, that means the opposite can happen too. When you're sedentary for too long, your brain and body don't get those boosts. They start thinking something is wrong with your overall bodily functions, and actually start to *disfunction.* Then, your body drags your mind through the resulting fog, making you feel tired, stressed, or even depressed.

That's what makes movement excellent medicine for our health! When we move our body, our mind becomes more alert, we become more energized, and our mood increases as serotonin, dopamine, and other chemicals are released. It's because of this that exercise is considered a "natural high" and is an easy way to stay not only physically healthy, but mentally, too.

Doctor Dean Ornish, a pioneer of lifestyle medicine, wrote a book titled *Undo It! How Simple Lifestyle Changes Can*

Reverse Most Chronic Diseases. In it, Ornish warns that "the combination of both sitting more than six hours a day and being less physically active was associated with a 94 percent increase in all cases of premature death rates in women, and a 48 percent increase in men, compared with those who reported sitting less than three hours a day and being most active" (Ornish, 2019). In other words, sitting is the new smoking.

But it doesn't just stop at bodily health; exercise helps our brains too. The brain is composed of billions of neurons that connect to one another through tree-like branches, forming an infrastructure that helps us experience every thought and feeling. Depression and long-term stress erode the connections between those neurons, which means that actively taking part in something that builds them back up can only be great for our mental health.

And the chemicals produced as a result of exercise – such as serotonin, dopamine, and gamma amino butyric acid, or GABA – are exactly what we need to achieve just that. In fact, these chemicals are the same ones targeted by common antidepressants and anti-anxiety medications. But exercise is a completely natural way to release these biological chemicals, making movement as good for our mood as it is for our body.

The mind-body benefits of fitness are outstanding; it's truly the greatest gift you can give yourself. In our seemingly increasing chaotic world, exercise can often be a safe refuge for our mind, body, and soul. And when you start to think about it that way, you give yourself the ability to start realizing it's less of a chore, and more of something that can be truly enjoyable, because there are so many different ways to get beneficial exercise without completely straining and draining yourself.

For example, did you know that simply walking or jogging twenty to thirty minutes a day could cut your chance of dying prematurely from things like heart disease in half (Andrews, 2022)? That's not to say you *need* to jog every single day, but it's incredible to see the beneficial proof of getting our bodies moving regularly!

According to Doctor Hamid in a review published in the *Journal of Aging Research,* exercise leads to longer life because it protects against cardiovascular diseases, type 2 diabetes, certain types of cancer, and neurodegenerative disease. A related study showed a 30-35 percent decrease in mortality and up to a 6.9-year increase in overall life expectancy for people who were regularly physically active.

Exercise is such a powerful medicine. I could write thousands of pages that show this to be true, but the truth is, those pages have already been written by so many incredible doctors and scientists! There are so many sources out there that can spell out exactly how and why our bodies love movement, and I encourage you to explore them. But when it comes to figuring out how exercising can help you achieve walking in STRENGTH and make your life the best it can be, the science behind the way our bodies work is less important than figuring out exactly how to make all that science work for *you.*

My Four Pillars of Exercise

Many people think that if they just run five miles a day, they'll be in peak health. While this kind of aerobic exercise is excellent for you, there are actually four distinct pillars of exercise that I believe every person needs to integrate into their workout routines in order to be as healthy as they can be.

The first is aerobic exercise, also known as endurance exercise or cardio exercise. The word "aerobic" is defined as "requiring oxygen," meaning this kind of exercise requires a higher amount of oxygen to circulate throughout your body to meet the demands of the physical activity being performed. So, exercises such as walking, jogging, running, swimming, cycling, or stair climbing fit this criterion, because they get your heart pumping and your lungs moving just a little faster.

The second pillar is muscular strength training. While aerobic exercise can help build some muscles, well-rounded strength training can help you become stronger and leaner throughout your body by building and maintaining your muscle tissue, improving your joint and bone health, and helping to decrease your risk of injury. Strength training can include exercises like lifting weights, working with resistance bands, or bodyweight exercise like push-ups, sit-ups, squats, or climbing stairs.

The third pillar is flexibility and mobility. Some flexibility can come from muscular strength training, but that type of training isn't truly enough to ensure that your body can move the way you need it to well into your later years in life. You may not believe that's true when you're young, but it will catch up to you as you age if you're not paying attention to increasing your flexibility and mobility while you're increasing your strength. Because the bottom line is if you aren't mobile, you can't exercise at all! Flexibility training can include exercises like stretching, yoga, tai chi, and Pilates.

Finally, my fourth (and extremely important) pillar of exercise is rest. This may come as a surprise, because resting isn't exercising, right? Wrong! Aerobic, strength, and flexibility exercises are all extremely important to your health, but they won't be nearly as effective if you don't give your body the time it needs to recover in between doing all those exercises. The reason is twofold: First, if your body can't recover from exercise, then it will be too exhausted to do more exercise later, meaning you won't be able to keep doing these things that are so healthy for you. But second (and more importantly), you don't actually build muscle and burn fat *while* you exercise. You do those things *while you recover,* after the exercise is done and even well beyond your workout. That's when your body has the chance to reboot, regenerate, and process all the exercise you did so that it can build up the muscles that you broke down while working out. Pretty incredible, huh?

The key to truly great exercise that's right for your body is getting these four pillars in perfect alignment. If you can determine the right doses of aerobic exercise, strength training, flexibility training, and rest for you, then you can achieve some incredible results.

Understand What Your Body Needs

Getting your four pillars of exercise in alignment is all about listening to your body and understanding what it needs. And that's what we've been practicing throughout this entire book so far!

So, what does your body need when it comes to exercise? The answer is: It varies. Sometimes you may need multiple days of rest. Sometimes you may need more strength training or more cardio or just lots of stretching to open tight areas. If you listen to your body closely (try a body scan!), it will speak to you and tell you what to target. If the muscles in one area feel weaker than others, try more flexibility and strength training that targets those areas. If your stamina and endurance throughout your day has taken a dip, try upping your aerobic exercise. And if you're feeling completely physically exhausted, then you know your body needs more rest.

Paying attention to the amount of stress your body is experiencing is also an excellent indicator of what workout might be best for you that day or week. For example, doing high-intensity cardio when your body's cortisol levels are high due to stress may not be the best thing for you. Instead, some gentle yoga might be just what you need to restore and strengthen your body. Don't think of it as a wasted day of exercise – think of it as giving your body exactly the exercise it needed at exactly the right moment.

And if you're having trouble reading exactly what your body needs, there are some incredible tools available to help with that these days! For example, the Oura Ring is a technological device that was founded and designed in Finland with the singular focus to improve the way humans live their lives. It's a lightweight titanium finger ring that contains 10,000 embedded sensors, including two infrared LEDs, an infrared detector, a gyroscope, three temperature sensors, and an accelerometer to measure your movements. When you wear your Oura Ring as they recommend, every morning it gives you an overall sleep score that expresses the quality of your sleep through a detailed analysis of the measurements it took while you were sleeping. It tells you not only how long you slept but how much deep sleep and REM sleep you had, how restless you might have been, and how ready you are for the day ahead, all largely based on measurements such as your heart rate variability and your resting heart rate. Having this insight can give you some *incredible* knowledge about your body and what kind of exercise it might be able to handle that day.

For me, the Oura Ring is a dream come true because it gives me so much important feedback. When the day starts, I can see my heart rate variability measurement and my resting heart rate so that I can understand how well I've recovered from my exercise the day before. Plus, this data has really helped me enjoy my sleep tremendously. It provides insight into how my choices made throughout the day before may have resulted in good or bad sleep that night, meaning I have the power to make better decisions daily.

There's nothing more inspiring than watching your biomarkers get better and knowing that your own behavior has improved everything, from your resting heart rate to your sleep quality. You can also share the information and data from your Oura Ring with your health practitioner if you need help interpreting it or want some more personalized guidance on how to improve your quality of sleep so you can improve the quality of your exercise.

I have learned so much about myself and can see just how beneficial good sleep is for energy levels, mental health, and the ability to joyfully engage in each and every day. And when we feel like joyfully engaging, it makes exercising all the easier and more appealing!

But if you're not quite ready to take on a new piece of technology, then using your journal to hand-write your data is also an excellent way to track yourself. Keep an exercise and activity log on the days you work out, and a rest log on the days you recover. Record all the exercises, stretches, and other activities you did, how long or intensely you did them, and then write down how you felt during, immediately after, and a few hours later. Do the same for the sleep you get at night by thinking about how restful (or un-restful) you were, and how tired or refreshed you feel the next day. Reflect back on this journal often to see how your daily activities, exercises, and rest all affect one another to track your status.

Once you start accurately reading your body's needs, you'll know what you need to focus on so that you can improve. From there, you can start to determine your exercise routine. But remember, your routine should ideally involve a healthy variety of the four pillars. And just as important: You should enjoy it!

No Commitment Without Enjoyment

If you've ever felt the exhilaration experienced after a run, or the mental clarity that comes after finishing a yoga class, or maybe the exhilarating post-workout pump that strength training can provide, then you've seen just how enjoyable exercise can be. It's true that these incredible sensations don't happen with *every* workout, but when they do, they remind us of exactly why we work out, and keep us coming back for more. So, the key to developing an exercise routine you stick with is to strive for that same level of rewarding enjoyment in every activity you do. In other words, you're much more likely to exercise when you enjoy the exercise!

When it comes to building stamina, strength, and flexibility over time, the most motivating thing you can do is have fun! Because if you're having fun, you're much more likely to keep working out and stick with your routine. If you try to force exercises into your workouts that you really despise, you're much more likely to skip the workout altogether for sheer lack of motivation to even try. That's why it's such a great idea to experiment with a variety of exercises and find the one that resonates with you the most.

I started running in college and have been doing it regularly for a long time. While I enjoy the occasional "runner's high," the true enjoyment I get from running comes specifically from having running partners. I've built beautiful, energizing relationships with these kinds of workout partners that I enjoy so much, it keeps me coming back. They are my truest and most treasured friends. They help me find deep encouragement and motivation to stay consistent. It's also the reason I love doing yoga, and love teaching yoga even more. When we're engaged in the activity together, the experience builds connectedness, and keeps everyone accountable and desiring to come back.

And I also reap benefits on my solo running or power walking days when I can be alone and in the moment, letting my creative thoughts and ideas surface. These are the days when I do a lot of my best thinking, which is also immensely rewarding and enjoyable! This learning came from experimenting with my workouts until I figured out what brought out the best in me, and then committing to doing more of it.

Experiment with a variety of exercises and find the one that resonates with you the most.

For someone like my husband, he reaps enjoyment in exercise through the competition of it. In his mid-fifties, he was consistent with his exercise thanks to how much he enjoyed doing CrossFit but had to stop due to other variables in life (as will naturally happen). But more recently, in realizing he needed to get back to exercising regularly, we decided to get a Peloton bike. And what a dramatic difference it has made for him! Not only are the trainer-guided workouts lively and fun, but he competes with our son, who has his own Peloton, to see who can get the best output, cadence, and resistance scores. The enjoyment he reaps from that motivation has kept him consistent while helping to rebuild his endurance, strengthen his heart, and grow stronger both physically and mentally.

Great exercise is all about balancing a healthy, well-rounded routine with those things you find the most joy in. I love changing up my exercise routines between high intensity training, jogging, and riding the Peloton on rainy days. But I could almost never do without the form of exercise that I take part in almost every single day: Yoga.

Let's Talk About Yoga

Yoga is one of the absolute best ways for people to take charge of and combat the stresses in their lives, while also adding the benefit of contributing to their mental and physical health. It's a wondrous practice that has had proven benefits for thousands of years, so I believe it's extremely deserving of its own space in the pages of this book.

I started practicing yoga in my forties, and now I not only practice it personally nearly every day, but I'm a nationally certified yoga teacher who loves helping others discover the incredible benefits of practicing. It's not just an exercise, though it certainly can be if that's how you'd like to think of it. But really, it has the potential to be a powerful lifestyle mindset that brings benefits beyond description – benefits that many people are unaware of.

According to the American Osteopathic Association (AOA, 2023), yoga's physical benefits include:

- Increased flexibility
- Increased muscle strength and tone

- Improved respiration, energy and vitality
- Weight reduction
- Cardio and circulatory health
- Improved athletic performance
- Protections from injury

Does that list look familiar? If not, I'll refresh your memory: It contains *all* the desired benefits that the four separate pillars of health can help you achieve. In other words, practicing yoga is one of the most well-rounded and balanced forms of exercise that you can do. I would even go so far as to say that if you choose to only partake in one form of exercise for the rest of your life, yoga would be your very best option to make sure you're getting all the types of exercise your body needs.

Not only is yoga physically incredible for you, but it improves your sleep, immunity, muscle recovery, and overall mental and emotional wellness. It has long been an activity known and recognized for calming and relaxing those who practice it, naturally making it an excellent choice for those who feel overly stressed. Because in addition to getting your body moving and eliminating a lot of muscle tension, yoga also asks you to be present in the moment. When you're focused on your breathing and body position, it's almost impossible to be overly concerned with other stressors in your life.

There are *so* many different forms of yoga and types of poses to discover and try – far too many for me to go through here. But there are some truly wonderful resources available in the form of books, magazines, websites, and videos that can help you discover which types of yoga are most enjoyable and beneficial to you. If you haven't experienced yoga, I'd love to introduce you to the joy of practicing yoga. Finding an instructor that fits your philosophy and style is well worth the time and will help you enjoy it to the fullest.

Action Points: ***Exercise and Move***	
Mindset	• Exercise doesn't have to be exhausting and grueling, but it does have to be a part of your journey to health. We only have one body, and we need to take care of it however we can! • Even just a little bit of movement on a consistent weekly schedule can make an incredible difference, so don't think of exercise as the enemy! Instead, find a way to enjoy it and have fun.
Skillset	• Understand and utilize the four pillars of health: Aerobic Exercise, Strength Training, Flexibility training, and Rest. • Understand what kind of exercise your body needs by listening closely to what it's telling you. • Experiment with a variety of exercises until you find the ones that are not only the most beneficial, but that you enjoy!

Action Points: Exercise and Move	
Skillset	• Keep track of your exercise and progress regularly so you can see where improvements need to be made. • Develop a consistent exercise routine based on what your body is telling you, the progress you're making, and the joy you feel!
Toolset	• A sleep measurement device such as the Oura Ring. • Other health devices and apps such as an Apple Watch can give you additional insight into what your body is experiencing and with your progress. • Journaling your exercise journey can be a good substitute for the above. • A variety of workout equipment such as a Peloton bike, treadmill, free weights, resistance bands, or a good pair of walking/running shoes can support your exercise journey. • Fitness groups and memberships to keep you accountable. • Yoga—in every shape and form! • Restful tactics (re-read Chapter 5 to refresh yourself!).

Remember every cell in your body loves movement of any kind! Doing simple daily exercises consistently keeps your heart strong, builds your fundamental muscle groups that power your body, and improves your overall flexibility and agility. Giving you the freedom to move confidently and fearlessly through life!

Now, let's "move" into our next powerful element of STRENGTH.

STRENGTH 7

Nutrify and Hydrate

Eating is an experience we get to enjoy immensely day after day. We derive satisfaction from all the delicious flavors, textures, and varieties of food, yet also reap the benefits and power of food fortifying our bodies. This together makes us fall in love with healthy eating. Isn't that thought amazing! Eating tantalizingly delicious real food gives us great pleasure and at the same time fuels and energizes the body and mind, and – also has the potential to prevent and even reduce disease.

"You are what you eat" may sound like some silly idiom, but there really is *so* much truth to it. So much truth, in fact, that I like to think of food as a very miraculous type of medicine. Even Hippocrates, the father of medicine, felt the same way when he was quoted to say, "Let food be thy medicine, and medicine be thy food" (Morrison, 2015).

This concept is quite simple, and yet, we as a society tend to dumb ourselves down regarding nutrition! We don't take time to truly understand and value what the food we eat does to and for our bodies, so without realizing it, we find ourselves putting whatever we want into our mouths, however much we want, and whenever we feel like it.

Yes, food is meant for our enjoyment. Selecting and preparing *good* food, I believe, is an art form and can be extremely satisfying on a regular basis. But we must remind ourselves that the primary, God-given purpose of food is to fuel and energize the body and mind, and it is often to be enjoyed surrounded by the people we love. The act of eating food is not meant to stress our body out or depress it. And yet, that's what much of the food we eat on a regular basis can do if we are not decisively intentional about what we choose to eat.

Joel Fuhrman, a nutritional scientist and a medical doctor specializing in cardiology, has said, "… doctors mostly prescribe medicines for conditions as a result of the toxic diet Americans are eating. That's like intentionally hitting yourself with a hammer and then going to a doctor to help you get better so you can keep hitting yourself with a hammer. In this case, the toxic foods we eat are the hammers" (Fuhrman, 2011). Now *that's* some food for thought!

But what exactly are toxic foods and how do they harm our mind and body? Most of the toxicity in our diet comes from highly processed foods. Highly processed foods are those that have been heavily altered from their original form and often contain artificial flavors and colors, as well as chemical preservatives and additives that, sadly, we and our children often become addicted to. These ingredients can be detrimental to our health both mentally and physically.

Research indicates that highly processed foods disrupt our gut increasing our risk of depression, anxiety, and mood disturbances, as well as increase our risk of heart disease, type 2 diabetes and some forms of cancer. These foods offer minimal, if any, nutritional benefits. Our grocery stores are loaded with these types of "foods". For example, packaged cookies are baked treats made with refined flour, sugar, and often contain artificial flavors and colors and processed oils. Corn chip snacks are coated with a flavored powder loaded with artificial ingredients and additives including highly inflammatory hydrogenated oils. Sodas are sugary carbonated beverages often containing high fructose corn syrup and artificial flavors. Most (but thankfully not all) items found in packaged foods or snacks provide little to no nutritional value.

If you are not sure how to identify these harmful ingredients, I highly recommend using the Yuka app, which is available for free. This user-friendly app allows you to simply scan the barcode of a food product and it provides you with insightful information. It rates the food product's health value based on its ingredients - giving you both the positives and negatives including any risky additives. My husband and my son-in-law love it and they make it a competition to see who can find the healthiest snacks. As a result, our pantries are stocked with tasty and reasonably healthy snack items.

However, highly processed foods and their additives are addictive, and it takes time to withdraw from these tasty, but empty foods. Yet in time and as you practice healthy lifestyle habits, you will recognize in yourself (and your children) the immediate effects these foods have on your mood and your sense of wellbeing. And eventually, you won't even *want them* on a regular basis anymore!

But if at this point in your journey, this looks like a mountain too high to climb, don't worry – you also don't have to go "cold turkey" on not eating foods you've become emotionally attached too. Treats *on occasion* do wonders for our soul and add joy to our celebrations in life.

So, let's focus on the power of nutrition as medicine. Let's focus on what a wonderful thing it can be by understanding what it does for us, how we can make it our friend, and how we can truly enjoy eating and sustaining ourselves in this way. Let's deep dive into the "N" in STRENGTH so we can discover all the ways that nutrition (and hydration!) can help us become the most healthy and vibrant versions of ourselves.

Food as Medicine

God designed food – real, natural food – to support our bodies to work at their highest potential to keep us healthy and well! In this way, you can think of food as medicine, and you can treat it that way when it comes to preventing disease and even reducing some diseases many of us experience in life. Food has the power to make us healthy or unhealthy in astounding ways!

In his book *Eat to Beat Disease,* Doctor William W. Li compares the effectiveness of food components to western medicine. He used sophisticated scientific models to test each one's various components, and found that almost every single time, the food beat out pharmaceutical drugs in effectiveness against things like high blood pressure and type 2 diabetes (Li, 2019). The right food has the power to do extraordinary things for our bodies, meaning we largely don't need all the western medications that many doctors these days are so eager to prescribe for their patients before considering how their diets can provide the medicine they need to feel better. Our society needs a whole new mindset for the 21st century in this regard.

Food is so transformative that we can use it to change our bodies on every level. For example, did you know that when you eat the wrong foods, your hormones can change, which can hijack your brain chemistry, which can then hijack the rest of your body? All by eating too many french-fries and drinking sodas!

There are even certain hormones that have been found to promote cancer and aging, such as excessive amounts of insulin or insulin-like growth factor (IGF) that are further exacerbated by the bad food we eat (Oxford Population Health, 2020). "The whiter the bread, the sooner you're dead," is a popular phrase often used to emphasize the potential health risk associated with consuming highly processed and refined white bread. Because the more of these harmful foods you eat, like sugar and white flour, the more you promote these hormones and increase the risk for diseases such as type 2 diabetes and cancer. A more positive popular saying is "The more you eat green, the more you get lean," because there are also healthy foods that can combat these bad hormones and processes – for example, leafy greens.

The right food has the power to do extraordinary things for our bodies.

Today, we have the unique opportunity in human history, with exponential advances in nutritional science, to gain the insight and power needed to truly use food as the very best form of medicine we could ever hope to prescribe ourselves. That's not to say that conventional medicine is not beneficial and often necessary, because it is. Yet we need to fully utilize what we have come so far in learning, specifically: which components of food make them healthy, which components don't, and the effects they can have.

I've come to realize the power behind this myself over the years as I've very closely examined what I eat and the results of eating it. My most memorable discovery actually came from eating spinach. When I was in my forties, I noticed that when I ate spinach, my energy level was maintained at a high capacity, with no mid-day crash. The more I substituted spinach for other foods, the truer this was. But that much of one thing can lead to burnout, so I gradually figured out that diversifying my leafy greens to include kale, collard greens, Swiss chard, arugula, and spring mix allowed me to maintain a high level of energy throughout my day, while still being satisfied with the food I was eating.

After experimenting with and learning from this simple alteration to my diet, I realized the possibilities were endless! Because if a few leaves from the earth could give me *that* much energy, then who knew what *all* the right foods could do for the rest of my body?

But What *Are* the "Right" Foods?

Much the same as choosing what type of exercise to experiment with and finding what works best for you, food has nearly endless options to choose from. There is an incredible variety of food that exists in our world, and it all has different effects on our body and mind. So, it really does come down to experimenting with those that work best for you and your goals. But I would like to at least break these options down into a few categories and lists that are important to understand and explore as a great place to start. From there, selecting your items at the grocery store becomes that much easier.

Fruits and Vegetables

There's an incredible amount of research and information that scientifically proves how beneficial diversified fruits and vegetables are to our body. And the key word here is "diversified." That's why, when it comes to this type of food, I always say remember to eat a rainbow of colors if you truly want all the benefits this wonderful food group has to offer. That's because foods of similar colors tend to contain similar elements.

For example, green vegetables, such as spinach and turnip greens, contain lutein and zeaxanthin, which may help shield against cancer and age-related diseases. Red foods like tomatoes, red bell peppers, and grapefruit contain lycopene, which may be important in fighting off heart disease. Blue and dark colored foods, such as blueberries and black beans, contain anthocyanins, which may also defend the body against cancer.

Additionally, our bodies thrive on many of the vitamins and minerals naturally found in fruits and vegetables. And many of them are antioxidants that can help reduce the risk of disease. Such essential vitamins and minerals include:

- Vitamin A
- Vitamin C
- Vitamin E
- Magnesium
- Zinc
- Phosphorus
- Folic Acid

Fruits and vegetables are also a good source of dietary fiber, with can help you feel full longer and support your digestive system. And because they're so low in fat, salt, and sugar, they can also help to lower your cholesterol and your blood pressure. If you regularly eat them, you can even be at a lower risk of developing type 2 diabetes or suffering a stroke, heart disease, and cancer – especially cancer of the bowel, stomach, and throat (Harvard School of Public Health, 2012). Fruits and veggies really are nature's medicine!

Some great types of vegetables to add to your diet are:

- Leafy greens, such as lettuce, spinach, kale, and collards

- Cruciferous, such as cabbage, cauliflower, brussels sprouts, and broccoli
- Marrow, such as pumpkin, cucumber, and zucchini
- Root, such as sweet potato and yam
- Edible plant stem, such as celery and asparagus
- Allium, such as onion, garlic, and shallot

Some great fruits to add to your diet are:

- Apples and pears
- Citrus, such as oranges, grapefruit, and lemons
- Stone fruit, such as nectarines, apricots, peaches, and plums
- Tropical, such as bananas, mangoes, and guava
- Berries, such as strawberries, raspberries, blueberries, and passionfruit
- Melons, such as watermelon, honeydew, and cantaloupe
- Tomatoes and avocados

You should strive to eat at least five servings of vegetable and two servings of fruit each and every day.

Protein

I'm not here to tell you that you need to have a total protein diet, but some studies are finding (and I'm personally experiencing) that as women, we *need* an ample amount of protein every single day for our bodies to function at their best.

Let's look at several of the important things protein does for your body by first looking at what happens without protein in your diet. Let's say you regularly start each day eating a high-carb breakfast (which many people inadvertently do because they don't realize that things like oatmeal and breakfast bars are high-carb and may have a lot of added sugars). What that does is spike your blood sugar early in the day, which leads to a crash and then a rollercoaster ride for the rest of the day. That crash can happen within the first fifteen minutes after eating, or a few hours later. Either way, you feel completely exhausted, and then you need more carbs or caffeine to get you back up, only to go right back down again.

If you make this kind of breakfast a regular habit, what happens in the long-term is that your body builds up insulin resistance. Eventually, this can lead to one of the many other diseases that we now know are connected at least in part to blood sugar dysregulation, such as type 2 diabetes, heart disease, increased cancer risk, and even dementia. Some experts are even calling dementia or Alzheimer's "type three diabetes!"

However, protein is an insulin buffer. By adding more of it to your diet, especially earlier in the day, you can keep those spikes and plummets at bay and keep insulin resistance from building over time and give your body the best chance of remaining healthy over the long term.

Next up are the wonders protein does for the hair, skin, and nails. I *know* many of us care about these features, and we may become more and more concerned about them as we age. Our hair becomes thinner, our nails get cracked and flaky, and our skin loses its luster and firmness. *But rather* than signs of age, these are all signs of simply not having enough protein in your diet. That's because your hair, skin, and nails are primarily *made* of protein, meaning they need as much of it as they can to keep looking good. So, if you're struggling with any of these issues, take a look at your protein consumption before you try some other chemical-based supplement that you likely don't need.

Other hormones in your body actually need protein in order to function correctly. For example, your thyroid gland, which is the central hub of your metabolism, requires the presence of the amino acid tyrosine to generate the necessary hormones that regulate your metabolism. Interestingly, proteins naturally break down into amino acids within the body. So it follows that having the right amount of protein in your diet can do wonders for boosting your metabolism and helping with weight management.

But the amino acids that come from protein play an even larger variety of roles throughout our body. For example, the neurotransmitters in your brain can't function correctly without sufficient amino acids from protein, which can lead to a decline in mental health. The amino acid phenylalanine is an especially essential component for neurotransmitters and the chemicals they produce, including epinephrine, norepinephrine, and dopamine. These chemicals are deeply associated with our fight-or-flight response, maintaining our blood pressure, and feeling happy.

Some excellent high-protein foods include:

- Lean meats such as chicken, turkey, and grass-fed beef and steak
- Eggs
- Greek yogurt and cottage cheese (without added sugar)
- Other cheeses, including feta, brie, gouda, mozzarella, Swiss, and parmesan
- Nuts and seeds, such as almonds, walnuts, chia seeds, and peanut butter
- Lentils and whole-grain products
- Soy products, such as edamame and tofu
- Seafood, such as cod, salmon, sardines, tuna, mackerel, crab, lobster, clams, and oysters

As you can see, protein plays such a huge role in our physical and mental health, so if you aren't getting enough of it in your diet, it's time to start! And you have some truly delicious options to give a try.

Omega-3 Fatty Acids

Although the human body can make most of the fats it needs from other food sources, the same does not apply for omega-3 fatty acids. They're considered "essential" fats because the body can't make them from scratch, and instead must ingest them from food. That's why it's so important to implement these types of food in your diet regularly!

But what, exactly, do omega-3 fats do for your body? They are critically important to maintaining healthy cells, and help create the hormones that regulate blood clotting, the function of artery walls, and inflammation. They also help to regulate genetic function. Due to all these factors, omega-3 fats have been shown to help prevent heart disease and stroke, and may even help control lupus, eczema, and rheumatoid arthritis, while also playing a protective role against cancer (Harvard School of Public Health, 2012).

When it comes to remembering how to choose the best sources of fish containing omega-3 fats, the acronym I like to use is S.M.A.S.H.:

- Salmon (wild-caught only!)
- Mackerel (Atlantic mackerel, preferably)
- Anchovies
- Sardines
- Herring

If you explore the website www.yourseafoodwatch.org, they provide some excellent lists of sustainable fish that are high in omega-3 fats, and will even let you know which ones are low in mercury, which is something very important to keep an eye on if you're consuming large amounts of seafood regularly.

"Brainfood"

You should now be well aware that taking care of your brain is just as important as taking care of the rest of your body!

For this and in general, I recommend the Mediterranean diet. The Mediterranean diet encompasses the same foods that a Harvard University study discovered promote healthier brain activity. (Harvard Health Publishing, 2021). These foods are:

1. Green veggies, especially leafy greens such as spinach, broccoli, and kale. They contain brain-health nutrients like vitamin K, lutein, folate, and beta carotene. They may also help slow cognitive decline. Avocados as well.
2. Fatty fish, which, again, are great sources of omega-3 fatty acids and healthy unsaturated fats. These have been linked to lower blood levels of beta-amyloid, a protein that damages the brain in those with Alzheimer's.
3. Berries, which contain flavonoids, the natural color pigments in things like strawberries, raspberries, and blackberries that help improve memory.
4. Black beans, which also contain flavonoids that improve memory, but they are also rich in soluble fiber and are a good source of prebiotics.
5. Extra virgin olive oil, which helps to reduce brain inflammation, improve moods, and assist with learning and memory.
6. Tea and coffee, which can offer a short-term concentration boost. But recent studies have shown that participants with a higher caffeine consumption actually scored better on mental functionality tests.
7. Nuts – walnuts in particular – are excellent sources

of protein and healthy fats that may also improve memory according to some studies.

The good news about this list is that it contains a lot of foods we've already discussed as being truly excellent for your overall health. So now, armed with all this knowledge about the best foods to implement for the healthiest diet, you have the power to put together some truly delicious and nutritious meals!

Treat Your Gut Right

In Chapter 3, we touched on the fact that your gut is like a magnificent tropical rainforest full of flora and bacteria, and how that microbiome has so much influence on everything you do. Eating a rainbow of colors helps to establish and build the diversified colonies of bacteria populating your gut, which helps support a highly functioning digestive tract. And the better your digestive track functions, the better the rest of your body and your brain operate.

But there are good microbes and bad microbes that exist in our digestive tract, each of them thriving on what we ingest in their own way. In the simplest of terms, "bad" foods, like highly processed foods and sugar, feed the bad microbes, and "good" foods feed the good ones. In general, the good microbes are the ones that serve as catalysts for producing good brain chemicals through that direct connection between your digestive track and your brain, so those are the microbes we want to make sure we're feeding properly. If we feed the "bad" ones too much, we feel sluggish, unproductive, irritated, depressed, and can't predict which way our mood might swing next.

Thankfully, ingesting something called prebiotics and probiotics can help to keep your healthy gut microbiome flourishing! These are compounds in food that induce the growth and activity of those beneficial microorganisms. The difference between the two? Prebiotics are soluble fibers that act almost like a fertilizer for your digestive system to help stimulate the growth of those healthy bacteria. Probiotics, on the other hand, are the specific bacteria found in certain foods that are similar to what's already naturally found in your gut, and they help you to repopulate your gut microbiome. Ingesting one without the other is a good start but ingesting them both together will *really* kick your gut health into gear!

There are some interesting (but tasty) foods that contain prebiotics and probiotics, and some examples include:

Prebiotics

- Garlic, leeks, and onions
- Kale
- Oats
- Chicory
- Asparagus
- Bananas
- Apples
- Flaxseed
- Cocoa

Probiotics

- Sauerkraut
- Kimchi
- Kombucha
- Yogurt
- Kefir
- Natto
- Cultured cottage cheese

You'll be amazed by what these simple additions to your diet will do for your energy, weight management, and mood. Eating these foods on a regular basis has personally shown me the importance of having these fermented foods in my diet. My energy stays strong, my skin stays smooth and free of any rashes or irritations, my digestive system works like a charm, and I bounce along with good moods and gratefulness most of my day. Wow, they're like super foods!

One of my favorite ones to take advantage of is sauerkraut. It's so simple to combine into soups, salads, and more. It brings flavor to any dish while simultaneously helping your body feel energetic and stable. Feel free to give some other prebiotics and probiotics a try to discover which ones you love best, then find ways to integrate them into your diet regularly!

Let's Talk About Hydration

No healthy diet could ever be complete without plenty of water! That's because it helps to prevent dehydration, which can cause unclear thinking, swings in mood, overheating, and even constipation and kidney stones.

The benefits of keeping dehydration at bay are pretty clear, but water is truly nature's wonder because of all the *other* incredible benefits it brings to our entire body – not just our digestive system. It can:

- Positively impact your immune function
- Increase your metabolism
- Help you maintain a higher energy level
- Lubricate and cushion your joints
- Protect sensitive tissues in the body
- Expel harmful wastes through urination and perspiration
- Make your skin look clearer, tighter, and brighter

Perhaps best of all, water has zero calories, so it can help to reduce calorie intake and manage body weight when it's substituted for other beverages in your diet.

The "correct" amount of water for any one person to drink per day is dependent on an array of factors such as age, height, weight, activity level, and even climate. But more is always better! And there's no better way to kick off your daily water intake than by drinking a full cup of water first thing in the morning on an empty stomach. It not only prepares your body and mind to drink more water throughout the day, but it can help kickstart your metabolism for the day too, which in turn can better aid in weight loss (Groth, 2021)! So put a full glass by your bedside every night, and when you wake up in the morning, reach for it and drink it down!

Drinking just enough water helps your bodily systems operate the way they need to.

Another great way to prompt yourself to drink more water throughout the day is to always have the option available. I like to fill up a stainless-steel cup or reusable bottle and take it with me everywhere, always keeping it within eyesight and reach so that I'm reminded to keep drinking. If you can refill this large cup or bottle a couple times in one day, you're off to a great start.

But even with this practice, I sometimes struggle with drinking enough water each and every day. So as a backup, I fill my fridge with water-dense foods – like watermelon! I almost always have watermelon around so that I can eat my water when I just don't feel like drinking it. It's such a hydrating fruit, and with the added bonus of being tasty!

Drinking just enough water helps your bodily systems operate the way they need to. But even *more* water can help those systems truly achieve their peak levels of performance! So, couple good hydration with good nutrition, and you're going to love the amazing energy and vibrance your body and mind give back to you every single day.

Control Your Triggers, Control Your Appetite

Here is where we really struggle with food – controlling our desire to eat. I'm not saying you shouldn't eat when you're hungry – food is fuel, after all! The problem is, in today's culture, the act of food consumption has morphed into an act of comfort and soothing, so we no longer eat solely because we need to fuel our bodies. We eat when we're stressed, sad, tired, bored, curious – you name it. Eating is associated with our emotions, with social interactions, with activities, and with holidays. It's embedded in our culture so deeply that it can be incredibly difficult to control what and how much we eat, because it's so socially acceptable – even expected – for us to eat, eat, eat.

And it becomes even more difficult to say no to food when a particular trigger that leads to eating kicks in. But I'm here to tell you that these triggers are not impossible to control, when you remember that *you* are in the driver's seat. It's all about being aware of what *your* eating triggers are, and having a strategic plan ready for when those triggers arise.

Personally, I've become aware that most of my triggers occur at night. That's the time when I peruse my pantry, searching for something salty and full of carbohydrates, but not because I'm hungry. Not usually, anyways. More often, there's some other reason behind that trigger, like boredom, cravings, or an emotion that I haven't dealt with properly.

When this happens and I catch myself in the pantry at 8 PM, I try to intentionally shift my mind to a different focus before I gobble up something. I find another outlet for myself, like starting my nightly routine earlier with activities such as reading, reviewing my joys of the day, and relaxing my mind and body with deep stretching. But that's a behavior I had to practice again and again to be able to utilize in times of need.

To figure out what your triggers are so you can start controlling your reactions to them, ask yourself these questions the next time you're hunting through the fridge between meals:

- Am I *really* hungry? Often times, you are actually thirsty and need hydration – you just don't realize it.
- Does my energy feel depleted, and will it be revitalized with food? Or is it something else? Like rest, comfort, time to reflect on my day, or another need.

Identify the reasons behind your desire to indulge, and next … go ahead and do it. I mean it! For the sake of figuring out how you *truly* feel about the food you eat, this is an important step in these early processes. Once you eat, ask yourself these questions next:

- Did I derive pleasure from eating that food?
- How do I feel an hour after eating? How about that night, or the next day?
- Am I glad I ate that food when I did? Or did I regret it later?

When you ask yourself these questions, you're looking at those eating habits you have every day that don't align with the idea of using food as fuel. Nearly everyone has them, even if they don't realize it right away.

I got into this practice of deterring myself from emotional eating by reminding myself that nothing controls me. How I eat and why I eat is my choice alone. I'm in the driver's seat – my emotions are not. I have all the power I need to make the right choices. Often, just reminding myself of this makes me feel grounded and free, which gives me the power to partake in much more mindful eating that I feel great about both in the short-term and the long run.

It all starts with being mindful of our triggers, slowing down to ask ourselves why they've prompted us to eat, and then refocusing our actions on some other activity. Do this enough times, and you'll no longer turn to food first when stress, boredom, or even those all-powerful cravings hit.

Though controlling your triggers to eat is a massively important part of getting your nutrition on the right track, there are tons more tips and insights that you can implement and practice in an effort to make healthier choices. One of my favorites is to slow down when eating a meal by deliberately stopping every two or three bites to put my fork down and chew, chew, chew my food mindfully. Not only will you digest better at this rate, but you'll feel fuller faster, and not to mention, you'll enjoy the flavors that much more.

Also, as you build your diet, don't do so with an "all or nothing" mindset. What I mean by that is, avoid telling yourself, "I'll *never* eat this," or "I will *only* eat that on weekends." You can allow yourself the freedom to eat anything you'd like. The key, however, is moderation. You can follow what I call the 90/10 principle: Ninety percent of the time fuel your body with highly nutritious food, and ten percent of the time allow yourself to thoroughly enjoy something that may not be quite as nutritious. If you'd like to eat a chocolate chip cookie, don't restrict yourself – go ahead and eat one. You don't need to banish yourself to a life of nothing but raw vegetables and bone broth.

Next, shop mindfully. One of the biggest reasons people eat large quantities of unhealthy food is because it's in their house, readily at their disposal. If you bring less bad food home after a grocery trip, you'll eat less of it. Pure and simple. Instead, stock your fridge with those foods that you've discovered both taste good, fuel you adequately, and don't cause any unwanted side effects like bloating, fatigue, or crashing.

In addition to stocking your kitchen with lots of healthy foods, try arranging your food in a way that makes it easier to make healthy choices. For example, fully prep your cooking station with all the healthy ingredients you need ahead of time. Also, when stocking your pantry and fridge, try putting the healthiest foods at eye-level, while arranging less-healthy snacks up higher or lower, or behind other products.

And don't forget to make your food flavorful! Contrary to popular belief, healthy doesn't have to mean bland. There are so many spices and herbs that can wake up the millions of receptors on your tongue to thoroughly satisfy your taste buds without having to dump salt on every dish. Some of these herbs can even give an added boost to your health, like turmeric, ginger, cumin, cinnamon, rosemary, parsley, peppermint, or chili powder. The list is endless!

You can also try something called intermittent fasting. This is when you restrict the window of time during each day that you eat all your food for the day. This prompts an extended period of metabolic reset so that your cells have a chance to essentially flush everything out and clean out your system before intaking food again, which can help with weight loss and management.

There are several different methods and varieties of time to experiment with when it comes to intermittent fasting, but one of the more popular is called the 16:8 ratio. What this means is that for sixteen hours of the day (including time spent sleeping), no food consumption takes place. Once that window has passed, then all food intake for the day must be completed within the remaining eight hours of the day before the sixteen-hour fast resumes. Because so much of that long window is spent overnight while sleeping, it's a very easy ratio to begin with.

Again, it's all about finding the methods, habits, and mindset that work best for you, and then being deliberate about the choices you make regarding those life-changing discoveries.

You can eat yourself to wellness,
or you can eat yourself to illness.
You have the choice and the power!

Keep Tabs on Consumption

As with most of the changes you've been making as you read this book, listening to your body and keeping track of what it's telling you is going to be one of the most effective ways to maintain your new nutrition choices. Your body speaks to you about everything you consume, and it's up to you to take note of what it's saying and become familiar with its patterns.

I can't say this enough! Notice what you're eating and how you feel after eating it. When you develop a habit of eating certain foods, you'll begin to experience consistent outcomes from consuming that food. This information is extremely helpful and through it, you'll be able to establish a diet that supports your body well, that you love to eat, and that gives you so much energy, it'll be coming out of your ears!

Keeping a journal of what you eat during the day can be very eye-opening. Not to mention, can help keep you accountable for what you're eating. So after your meal or snack, take some notes on how the food made your body and mind feel. This habit will also help you to see just how much and what kinds of foods you're consuming on a daily basis, and better determine where you need to make changes. But remember, show yourself grace! Don't journal your food with judgement, and instead, think of it as giving yourself freedom to be as intentional as you can about what you eat.

After you consistently journal about the foods you eat and the reactions they cause for a couple of weeks, you'll very easily be able to see which foods leave you feeling ready to conquer the world, and which ones make you want to crawl into bed and sleep. From there, you have the power to essentially hack into your own body by giving it exactly what it needs to perform at its very best.

Remember: You can eat yourself to wellness, or you can eat yourself to illness. You have the choice and the power!

And most importantly, focus on the joy of eating. Enjoy every aspect of it – including all the wonderful tantalizing flavors, textures, and aromas. Enjoy the energy all those foods produce for you and the happy moods that come as a result.

Action Points: *Nutrify and Hydrate*	
Mindset	• Think of food as medicine! The right foods have the power to heal your body and prevent so many ailments and diseases. • Mindfully eat. Take time to enjoy the entire eating process, engaging all your senses, being aware of the taste, texture, and aromas, as well as the act of chewing and swallowing. Also, think about how those specific foods are revitalizing your body and mind. • Perseverance – make up your mind to stick with it. Remember that after only a few short weeks of consistently eating healthy, you will begin to crave healthy foods over unhealthy foods. In fact, junk food and snacks will be repellent to you.

Action Points: Nutrify and Hydrate	
Mindset	• Think of food as your fuel that charges and recharges your metabolic system, keeping all cylinders firing at highest capacity.
Skillset	• Research and experiment with the variety of healthy foods that are available to you. • Take time to discover what the right foods are, and then be deliberate about integrating them into your diet. • Determine which foods deliver the best sustainable energy level for you! • Identify and understand the triggers that cause you to eat emotionally, including recognizing how certain foods make you feel. • Notice your eating patterns. When you discover an unhealthy emotional pattern, then refocus your attention on something else: What else soothes you, excites you, comforts you and do that instead. • Set up your surroundings while you're preparing and eating in a way that creates peace and joy, whether by yourself or with others.

Action Points: Nutrify and Hydrate	
Skillset	• 90/10 principle – Ninety percent of the time fuel your body with highly nutritious food and great movement. Ten percent of the time allow yourself to enjoy a little bit of something that may not be quite as nutritious.
Toolset	• This list can be nearly endless because there are so many healthy, well-rounded foods to choose from! Start with vegetables, fruits, protein, omega-3 fats, and brainfood. • Eat foods that span the colors of the rainbow throughout your day to reap the benefits of essential vitamins and minerals. • Integrate some prebiotics and probiotics into your diet regularly. • Use the Yuka App to see the health value of a food product before buying it. • Use your journal to keep track of your eating habits and your reactions to certain foods. • Explore recipes that integrate the healthy foods you love, remembering to use an array of herbs and spices to make them tasty instead of sugar or salt.

Action Points: *Nutrify and Hydrate*	
Toolset	• Water! Drink a big glass first thing in the morning and always carry a full water bottle with you to drink throughout the day.

Healthy food not only fuels and energizes the body and mind but also prevents and reduces certain diseases. As you continue to nutrify and hydrate by applying the mindsets, skillsets, and toolsets described in this chapter, you'll notice positive changes in your body – in how you look and most importantly in how you feel! And in no time at all, you will be well on your way to becoming the most healthy and vibrant version of yourself!

8 STRENGTH

Goal-Set with Grace

You might be wondering how setting goals has anything to do with being healthy. Goals aren't leafy greens. They're not an aerobic workout. They aren't a good night's sleep. So where do goals even fit into the bigger picture of discovering how to live in STRENGTH? The answer: goals will help you make what you want for yourself a reality.

Think about it this way: goals are a tool. They help you put what you want to achieve into clear focus. Having written goals keeps you accountable, motivated, and on target. Also, the action steps you develop along with each of your goals provide you with the roadmap on how you are going to get there.

Goals can be *incredibly* powerful motivators for achieving great things. But believe it or not, there are right ways and there are wrong ways to think about and set goals. Though the goal of developing transformative lifelong holistic habits is a great place to start, the reality is, it's such a broad goal that without taking time to break it down, refine it, and better understand it, it's going to be really tough to stick with.

And that's where the "grace" part of this chapter comes in. Goal setting is an ambitious task. Many people don't do it at all because they're afraid of failing to reach their goals. But if we approach the process with grace and kindness toward ourselves, and with enthusiasm for what we can achieve, we have so much more power to get there!

Personally, I love setting goals. I am a lifetime goal-setter, one of those people who loves to come up with something, think about how it would feel to attain it, and then do everything I can to get there. And I hope to ignite in you a love for setting goals as well! Goals that are motivated by faith, infused with grace, and that unleash freedom, not fear or judgement.

When you understand the best way to set achievable goals, and you approach the process with grace, the possibilities for what you can achieve are truly endless.

Why Set Goals?

Would you be surprised if I told you that setting goals isn't always about achieving them? It's not necessarily the end product we're looking for. Instead, setting goals is about establishing a *system of change that leads us to becoming the person we want to be.* The goal does provide a finish line, but *all the positive changes that occur on the way* to that line are what matter most.

So then why even set goals, instead of just enacting the changes we want? Because again, goals can be exactly the motivator we need to get started and actually stick with those processes. And then, once we do reach a goal, we already have some incredible habits in place that will help us to set and work toward another goal, and then another, and another.

Goals can also provide increased focus and productivity, boost motivation, and increase commitment. And they allow us to learn from and celebrate ourselves. Each step in the right direction is cause for celebration! And each failure is an opportunity to learn how to work harder and smarter. In that way, there's really no failing at all – only readjusting and continuing onward. Having that mindset about goals makes them a lot less overwhelming.

But remember, personal growth involves change, and we all know change is uncomfortable; as humans, we tend to avoid change as much as possible, because there's safety and comfort in familiarity. So, setting goals can help get us into the mindset of being more comfortable with enacting change in our lives.

And remember, every time we set a goal, we are also exercising faith by responding to our inner convictions and deep desires divinely fashioned by God. With determination, endurance, and God's help (fueled by our trust in Him), we can achieve anything. But we don't have to have giant buckets of faith to accomplish goals; we just need to know we have a BIG God who can do anything and is for us. Instead, our job is to prayerfully establish a plan whereby those big things can happen.

I like this definition of success from author Tommy Newberry: "Success is the deliberate, measurable pursuit of prayerfully chosen written goals." Achieving success through setting goals means having an intentional approach to life that ensures you are a faithful steward of your God-designed gifts and talents. This desire compels me to grow and develop myself. Finding success doesn't depend on the other circumstances of my life, but on the internal condition of my soul (Newberry, 2007). So, for me, using goals to find success looks like this:

1. Praying about my goals and earnestly seeking God in his truth before I set them
2. Aligning my goals with my deep beliefs, core values, and principles
3. Putting my goals in writing for accountability
4. Taking measurable action to achieve my goals

Setting the right kinds of goals helps us have a target to head toward, and a strategy for getting there. It also pushes us to move forward without overwhelming us. It's all about thinking big and then breaking down our goals into smaller components. From there, we can develop and establish habits by *creating a system* to keep improving. And when we reflect on and review our goals and habits regularly, we can gain clarity on our progress and what might need to change.

Do It the SMART Way

So how do we set these truly helpful, motivating, and achievable goals I speak of? By being SMART about it!

SMART goals were developed by George Doran, a consultant and former Director of Corporate Planning for Washington Water Power Company in 1981. He and his colleagues researched and wrote an article about *creating a system* whereby management goals and objectives were more achievable, and they came up with a memorable acronym detailing that all goals should be made:

- **S**pecific
- **M**easurable
- **A**ttainable
- **R**ealistic
- **T**ime bound

Over the decades, many people the world over have found these elements to be applicable not just to management and leadership goals, but to nearly *any* type of goal one wishes to set out to achieve. That's because the SMART technique requires you to truly break down the elements of your bigger goals into smaller goals that you can achieve and build from. It stipulates that each time you set a goal, you should ask yourself these questions:

- Is this goal **specific**? What am I trying to achieve? Why am I doing this? Who will be involved in me achieving this? Be as detailed as possible.
- Is this goal **measurable**? If so, how will I measure what I'm doing, or the progress I'm making? If it's not measurable by numerical data, how else will I assess my achievement?
- Is this goal **attainable**? Do I have the right tools to reach my goal? If not, what do I need? Be honest with yourself about your available time, energy, and income.

- Is this goal **realistic**? Can I *actually* meet the goal I've set? Or do I need to rethink the size and scope of my goal to be more realistic? Again, think about what you can feasibly achieve with where you currently are in life.
- Is this goal **time bound**? What is the timeline for reaching my goal? What deadline will I give myself to accomplish it? Work backwards, starting with your final objective, and create a checklist of steps needed to get there.

The more detailed and specific you are in answering each of these questions, the clearer picture you'll have of what your goal entails, what you want your end result to be, and all the requirements of getting to that stage. And yes … *write it all down!* A recent study of more than 250 participants indicated that you are 42 percent more likely to achieve your goals just by writing them down (Hyatt, 2022).

Let's look at an example of SMART goal setting. Saying, "My goal is to move and exercise more," is a good starting point, but it's vague, hard to measure, and doesn't provide a sense of time. That's going to make it hard to stick with and to know if you're even working toward it in a helpful way. Instead, try something like, "My goal is to go to a yoga class at least twice a week starting November 1st through March 1st."

This goal is:

- Specific: It states exactly what the activity is, and who is involved.

- Measurable: Attending yoga twice a week is a measurable factor.
- Attainable: It spells out the tools you need to accomplish it, which are access to a yoga class and a time to attend.
- Realistic: It does not overwhelm by aiming for yoga every single day. Practicing yoga twice a week is a much more realistic goal to achieve.
- Time Bound: Not only does it establish a number of days per week, but a finite window of time in which to achieve the goal.

The beauty of a goal like this is that you will know exactly whether or not you've achieved attending at least two yoga classes per week by the time you get to the end of that four-month window. If you've achieved it, you can build from it and set a larger goal. If you didn't achieve it, you can reflect on why that was, readjust as needed, and try again.

See how much power there is in breaking big dreams into smaller, more definable, more achievable goals? It keeps us so much more accountable and gives us the ability to continue creating and achieving goals again and again, until we're right where we've always wanted to be.

Accountability is a *huge* factor in you reaching your goals. Accountability to others you choose to involve is great, but accountability to *yourself* is even more important. When we follow through with ourselves, with others, and with God, and we achieve what we set out to do, it builds a sense of personal integrity and accomplishment that is so incredibly motivating!

A great place to start in setting your SMART goals is to create at least one goal for every element of STRENGTH in this book. I know we haven't gotten through all of them yet, so for now, go back through the previous chapters and create a goal related to the habits you want to see form in relation to that chapter. Remember, consistency is what we want to establish when we set these goals, so that we can better form those healthy habits on the way to becoming the best versions of ourselves. So, think about that and *enjoy the process*!

The Importance of Measurement

If you don't know what kind of progress you're making, then you have no idea whether or not you're actually working toward the goal you've set. And if you can't see that progress, you're much less likely to stick with the goal. That's why thorough measurement, as well as regular review and reflection on that measurement, is such an important part of this process.

It's important to write down all the details of your SMART goals, because there's a good chance that your goals will change as you work your way through them. That's just part of life! Things change, elements get in the way, or progress is even sometimes made faster than you anticipated. So, revisiting your goals and adjusting them is an important part of the measurement process. Make sure you read over them regularly!

Depending on the nature of your goal, there is an abundance of tools at your disposal for measuring your progress towards it. My favorite tools are the ones that give me progressive data I can look at and learn from. For example, if you have a specific goal related to sleep and rest, you might consider purchasing something like the Oura Ring or a WHOOP sleep tracker. I've used them both and they are both excellent!

If your goals are related to weight loss, a tool like a Withings scale is an excellent way to track your bone weight, your body mass index (BMI), your water weight, your muscle mass, and your body fat. This is all essential, progressive, and measurable information that you can acquire on the way to learning your patterns, so you can make adjustments as needed.

Even that Apple Watch, Fitbit, or Garmin watch on your wrist can be an excellent tracker for your physical measurements and progress! These tools can give us so much incredible insight into your everyday activities, but just be sure to visit their associated apps or websites so you can see all the data laid out in front of you and understand what kind of measurable progress you're making.

These kinds of tracking devices are extremely important to measuring progress, and it's amazing what we have access to these days! So, I highly recommend researching the tracking devices that are useful to your specific goals. They will give you the ability to measure important aspects of your health and to help you attain your goals.

Celebrate your success!

Another great option for biological measurement is getting your blood work done. I get mine done every six months to see and understand certain parameters of my health and how they're changing. I like to see my patterns, so I'm aware of the progress I'm making or if I'm maintaining the same level of health. When you sense something could be off, bloodwork like this can give you an important level of insight.

The last thing I always say is *so* important is to celebrate your success! Especially right now, in these beginning stages of working your way to living in STRENGTH, it's so important to celebrate every bit of progress you have made toward your goals. And you can't celebrate that progress if you don't measure it.

None of us reach our big goals overnight, but we see progress over time as we make small incremental changes. And over a longer period of time, these lifestyle changes become habits that transform us. A baby step in the right direction can turn out to be the biggest step in your life. Reaching a small goal is just as important as reaching a big goal because it means we're on our way to becoming a new person – a person we can't wait to keep celebrating.

Action Points: Goal-Set with Grace	
Mindset	• To cultivate healthy habits, it is essential for us to establish measurable and attainable goals. • These goals are incredible motivators, self-esteem boosters, and productivity enhancers. • What matters most when working towards your goals are all the positive changes that occur on the way. This can be more important than achieving them. • Always set your goals with grace. Be kind to yourself during this process. • There's really no failing at achieving your goals – only readjusting and continuing onward.
Skillset	• Every goal should be a SMART goal in order to give you the greatest chance of achieving it: Specific, Measurable, Attainable, Realistic, and Time bound. • Measure your goals thoroughly and consistently to know what kind of progress you're making. • Write each goal down and read through and reflect on your goals and your progress regularly.

Action Points: Goal-Set with Grace	
Toolset	• Your core values and beliefs will help you figure out how to align your goals with who you truly are. • Your vision board can be an excellent resource for figuring out exactly what goals you want to set. • Your journal will be necessary for writing out your SMART goals and tracking them. • Tracking devices like the Oura Ring, WHOOP, Withings Scale, and activity watches are great for measuring your physical progress. • Getting your bloodwork done regularly can give you even more biological insight into your health journey.

Goals are such an important part of living in STRENGTH because on the journey to betterment, we often find ourselves thinking about what we *should* be doing instead of focusing on and going after our truest core values and desires. Breaking down your goals in a way that makes them authentic to yourself and your future vision means you are truly setting goals for *you*.

So, when you start to think, "I *should* be doing what everyone else is doing," just remember that no one knows what you really need and really desire, so "should" is irrelevant. All that matters is that you are reaching a goal that you want to reach, and it doesn't matter if someone else values that goal. All that matters is that you do what you want to achieve and move towards who you want to become – all for the higher good. You are designed to flourish in your own unique ability and purpose and your goals can help you get there!

9
STRENGTH

Thrive in Your Community

Take a moment to think: When was a time you felt truly alive? Now, consider how much of that feeling came from being with the people around you. Thus far throughout this entire book, we've been discovering all the healthy ways to empower ourselves to authentic, optimal wellbeing. We've talked about how our focus and effort need to be directed toward cultivating our best health and establishing goals in our day-to-day journey.

Now we will shift gears a little to talk about the "T" in STRENGTH – *thrive* in your community – and how the people outside ourselves are so important to this process. But let me explain why community, and more specifically, why *spending time* with community is so incredibly beneficial to our growth as people and to our own health.

"Community" can mean and look like a lot of different things to different people. It can refer to family, friends, colleagues, neighbors, and more. It can be large and varied, compact and tight-knit, or any size and shape in between. That's the beauty of community, really. It's what we make it and what we reap from how we've made it. In that way, our communities, and the joy we experience from interacting with them, are as unique and varied as we as individuals are.

But some people have recently claimed that the current generation is the loneliest to have ever lived on Earth. Just think about that! In a day and age when the world population is the largest it's ever been, and connections can be made around the world with the click of a button, people feel lonelier than ever. Why is that?

I believe it's precisely *because* that's how so many modern connections are made: Through a screen rather than face-to-face. God didn't design humans to be lone wolves; He gave us our miraculous emotional intelligence so that we could have meaningful interpersonal relationships that enrich our lives and stimulate our happiness. And those effects just can't be achieved through 280 characters on X or a thirty-second video on TikTok. To be truly healthy of mind and soul, we need real, live interaction with the community that fills us with joy. And we need to be as deliberate about building those habits into our lives along with all the other healthy habits we're on our way to building.

COVID-19 and Community

The year 2020 was an incredibly difficult time for people all over the world. With the COVID-19 pandemic climbing to its highest infection rates, cities were shut down, sheltering in place took effect, and we were all made to temporarily become those "lone wolves" we were never meant to be. It was a wide-scale social shutdown the likes of which many of us will likely never experience again in our lives. Thank goodness!

To be truly healthy of mind and soul, we need real, live interaction with the community that fills us with joy.

That isolation resulted in significant psychological consequences for many people. It has caused ongoing anxiety, panic, depression, obsessive compulsive symptoms, post-traumatic stress, insomnia, and even digestive problems (because as we know, your mind and your gut are connected). Prolonged periods of isolation, sometimes even as short as several days, can have long-term mental and physical effects that can take *years* to recover from.

I witnessed my sister and my brother fall victim to isolation, and I watched the consequent down-spiraling negative effects on their health. That's because the removal of relationships from our lives eliminates the conditions we need for essential development of our personal identity. This can in turn cause us to become irrational, detached, angry, and sad.

Now that we're on the other side, we realize how much we truly need each other. Without face-to-face interaction on a consistent basis, we as individuals, families, and communities all suffer. Prioritizing face-to-face connection and community in our lives is foundational to living in true health.

Good Health Means Good Relationships

There has been so much developing research over the last few decades (and especially over the last few years, due to the pandemic) about the importance of community. One of the most impressive and eye-opening has been a study done by Harvard University released in 2017 that took place over the span of eighty years!

Scientists began tracking the health of nearly 300 Harvard students during the Great Depression (1929 through the late 1930s), with the goal of "[revealing] clues to leading healthy and happy lives" (Mineo, 2017). Over time, that same study expanded to look at the lives of the students' spouses and children. They studied their health trajectories, careers, marriages, and various life triumphs and failures. During those eight decades and hundreds of lives looked at, the researchers concluded one very important and common factor between all of them: "… our relationships and how happy we are in our relationships has a powerful influence on our health … taking care of your body is important, but tending to your relationships is a form of healthcare too."

They found that the people who were the most satisfied with their interpersonal relationships at age fifty were the physically healthiest group of people by age eighty. That's because healthy and consistent relationships, more so than money, fame, or success, help to delay mental and physical decline. The study even claimed that relationships are "better predictors of long and happy lives than social class, IQ, or even genes."

Isn't that incredible? Just imagine: You could potentially live a longer and healthier life if you consistently surround yourself with people – people to love you and people to receive your love.

When I was experiencing all the difficulties with my sister's and brother's declining health, my community was a huge place of comfort and strength. Without that support, I don't know that I would have come out intact on the other side. When we go through these kinds of struggles and chaos in our lives, having a supportive community makes a huge difference in how well we cope and how well we recover from that rough season. And sometimes, our community, and the even stronger bonds we forge with them can be *the biggest gift to result from the suffering.*

For me, having close friends who supported me was endlessly valuable as I spent much time traveling back and forth across the country to donate my bone marrow to my brother, and to support him and his wife. It was physically taxing, not to mention, emotionally chaotic. Trying to process that entire experience while away from my own life and my three young children would not have been possible without the support of my friends encouraging me and helping take care of my children.

But our community doesn't just make the hard times more bearable. It has the power to make the good times even more wonderful. I like running, but I would never have become such an avid runner if it wasn't for one of my closest friends encouraging and challenging me. My church community, yoga training community, family, fitness class community, and my closest friends (who I've walked through life with) have all contributed beautiful memories that I will cherish forever, as the priceless gifts they are.

Yes, these relationships are investments, because time and commitment were (and still are) crucial to developing them. Over the years they've required lots of forgiveness, grace, and honesty. But I wouldn't trade all the work I put in for anything. That's how much I value the community I've worked so hard to build throughout my life.

Just like other habits, developing strong community and relationships is a discipline.

Of all the research, articles, and documentaries about those entering their later seasons of life, the one common regret many of them share is about not spending enough time with family and friends or developing closer relationships with the people in their lives. They don't regret not making enough money, or not traveling the world, or even not always eating healthy and exercising regularly. Above everything else, they most regret not having spent more time with the people they love and not cherishing the time that they did have with them.

If you don't want to find yourself with those same regrets when you reach your last season of life, then you *must* put the work in now. You *must* make developing and fostering your community a habit – the same way we've worked on making so many other things a habit up to this point. I know you can do it! God built each one of us to have the desire and need to connect with those around us. If we just take the time to listen to those needs, we have the power to use them to find true joy and purpose in our lives.

How to Find and Foster Your Community

Whether you're sixteen, thirty-two, or seventy-seven years old, there's always a way to find a community that can help you thrive. Sure, for some age groups, like those who are still in school, it's a little easier; when you're in forced proximity with similarly aged and like-minded people, there's more opportunity to forge relationships with them. As we become adults, we can decide to spend more time in isolation or to choose the social events and gatherings we want to partake in, which means it becomes more difficult to find our tribe. But it's never impossible!

Start by closely examining those hobbies and activities you enjoy doing. Maybe it's reading great books, practicing yoga, or cooking healthy meals. Make a list of all the activities you enjoy. Then, make a list of all the possible social aspects of those activities. For reading, it could be book clubs or live author readings. For exercise, it could be gym or community classes. For cooking, it could be live group lessons or shopping at fresh farmers markets. These are all excellent places to start looking for meaningful relationships that could enrich your life.

Though filling your life with a variety of healthy communities and relationships is important, so is spending time fostering the interpersonal relationships you already have, and that you would like to make stronger. These are the people you want to have the closest and most meaningful bonds with when you start to enter those later seasons of life. They might be family, spouses, or close friends. If they are important to you, then it's important to prioritize them.

Just like other habits, developing strong community and relationships is a discipline. It's a habit that's formed as you make small, incremental changes to carve out time for people in your life on a regular basis. If you can do that, then you will be on your way to making your relationships the highest priority in your life and reaping all the health benefits that come with doing so.

One great way to start is by realizing the importance of taking your relationships off screens and social media, and making time for real, face-to-face interaction. And you don't have to always be planning long weekend getaways or hosting grand parties to accomplish this. Even just carving out an hour a week to meet up for a cup of coffee, take a walk through the neighborhood, or have another family over to play and share a simple meal together can provide so much ground for meaningful connection to occur.

However, consistency is key here. The more time you make for others, the stronger your relationship will be. For example, meeting up with old college friends once a year is nice, but it's hard to foster a truly deep and meaningful relationship with them if you only get a chance to catch up for a few hours once every 365 days. So, find ways to make time for them in the in-between, too.

Also understand that conflicts are bound to arise in any relationship. That doesn't mean it's not healthy, or that the relationship isn't developing, or that you're just not meant to make this person a part of your community. It means you're human! Sometimes we need some messy conflict in our relationships with people in order to grow relationally, improve our communication skills, and learn how to understand someone who sees things differently than we do.

This is a great opportunity to practice creating SMART goals for yourself! Start by thinking about those relationships in your life that you'd like to work on making stronger and more meaningful. Or start by thinking about all the ways you'd like to find a community that's meaningful to you.

From there, set your first SMART goal. Remember, that means the goal must be: Specific, Measurable, Achievable, Realistic, and Time bound.

For example, if you're actively seeking grow your community or tribe, your SMART goal could be something along the lines of "I want to attend one women's event at church or one kick-boxing class per week for the next twelve weeks, and I will introduce myself to at least three people during every class." Remember, it's all about starting with smaller, easier-to-achieve goals that will eventually lead to larger sweeping habits and changes.

Action Points: Thrive in Your Community	
Mindset	• The community we create and foster is perhaps the most important factor in our long-term wellness and health. So, our relationships deserve just as much time and attention to forming good habits associated with them as all other health habits do.
Skillset	• Being deliberately proactive and consistent with either seeking out your community or working on enhancing the relationships you already have is key. • You can build and improve these relationships by making them in-person and occur regularly, as well as by working on mindful communication, which takes honesty, respect, and an understanding that we humans are flawed – and that's okay!
Toolset	• All of the hobbies and activities you take part in regularly and enjoy doing are great arenas for fostering new community relationships. Explore them thoroughly to meet new people!

Action Points: Thrive in Your Community	
Toolset	• SMART goals will help you determine exactly how you want to improve your relationships, and what you need to do to get there. • The internet and social media *can* be a good place to research where you might find like-minded people who can become your tribe, but don't rely on it too heavily for forging your relationships. Get out there and do it for real!

Finding and thriving in community and fostering our most important relationships strengthen and fortify our lives. It not only fulfills our unique purpose of building up others around us but also greatly enhances our health and wellbeing.

10 STRENGTH

Hone Your Healthy Habits

Look how far you've come! You've opened your mind and your heart to new concepts and ideas. Chances are, you've gained insight into yourself, your beliefs, your values, and your habits. In all likelihood, you've identified certain habits that are not benefiting you anymore, and you're excited to replace them with empowering new ones. Moreover, perhaps you're already actively working on establishing those empowering new ones! All that work is to be congratulated – and know that I'm cheering alongside you all the way! And just like a runner racing to the finish line, we want to finish strong – because this final letter in STRENGTH is essential in making these habits a regular and consistent part of your life.

"H" is the last habit in STRENGTH and stands for "honing your healthy habits". It's all about putting everything you've learned together and truly turning it into a complete lifestyle change for yourself. And this is accomplished by understanding how to make these changes into habitual patterns you will follow for the rest of your beautiful life!

I want to start by reminding you why we've created these healthy habits and why you are working at implementing them into your daily lifestyle step by step, day by day:

- Our lifestyle habits greatly impact the level of sickness and disease in our wellbeing, whether physical, mental, or spiritual.
- Our lifestyle habits also have great potential to *prevent* sickness and disease..
- Our lifestyle habits can make a *huge* positive difference in our wellbeing – delivering real steady energy, a well working metabolism, focused clear thoughts, and healthy emotions.

Along with that, your own personal unique *why* that you created early on in this book is a big part of your motivation to hone your healthy habits. As you hone your STRENGTH habits, they will become integrated into your lifestyle and become part of who you are.

How Habits are Formed

At this point, this information is a refresher, but repetition is a great way to remember important things! And the concept of how a habit is formed is similar: A habit is a behavior that has been repeated enough times to become automatic. In other words: Repeat, repeat, repeat! When habits are automatic, we use less mindful energy and effort to perform them, which is the ultimate "purpose" of habits – to do something instinctively and more easily.

It's encouraging to remember that even tiny behavioral changes have the power to bring about remarkable results when they're consistently repeated. However, that goes for both good and bad habits. So that means you must work on repeating and reinforcing the good ones!

Still, we all know that it's very difficult to just quit doing a "not so good" habit cold turkey. That goes against the very nature of an established habit, after all. So, it's better to think of honing your habits as reinforcing a new or good habit so that it eventually replaces the old habit.

To implement a useful mindset of replacement over deletion, I always like to recommend "The Four Laws of Behavior Change" as introduced and described by James Clear in his book *Atomic Habits* (2018). It's a simple and straightforward set of rules to follow to build these better habits that will be replacing our old ones. They are:

1. Make it obvious.
2. Make it attractive.
3. Make it easy.
4. Make it satisfying.

To make something obvious, you want to keep it at the front of your mind. Often, that can mean keeping it in front of your *eyes*. In other words, don't hide the healthy fruits and vegetables you're trying to eat more of in the very back of the fridge. Make them the first thing you see when you open the refrigerator door. Arrange your pantry so that the lower nutritional snacks are almost unreachable. Likewise, keep the healthier foods within easy reach. If you are trying to increase your daily intake of water, then always keep the water bottles you use clean and easily accessible. One thing I do is to also keep my lemon essential oil right next to the refrigerator. That way it is easy and quick for me to add one drop in my water bottle each time I refill it and I'm good to go! Make your habits as easy as you can for yourself by making them obvious to see and easy to access.

To make something attractive is pretty self-explanatory: Make the habit you're trying to implement something you actually want to try doing. *Make it appealing to you.* For example, if you're trying to read more books instead of watching so much TV, then choose books that you know will likely appeal to you – whatever is a "page turner" for you. My husband doubled his daily water intake (and reduced his soda intake) by simply buying an 18-ounce canopy green Yeti Rambler® water bottle with a chug cap. Because he likes the way it looks, how it keeps his water cool and clean, and how easy it is to hold using the top handle, I find him carrying it all around with him and drinking from it all day long!

To make something easy is again, self-explanatory: Don't make the new habit difficult to achieve. Going back to the fruit and vegetable example, don't decide that your new habit will be to eat more wildly exotic fruits and vegetables that are difficult to find in a grocery store. Select produce that's easy to find and purchase. You will most likely stick to your healthy habits when you make them something you can easily put into practice.

Making something satisfying is different from making something attractive. When you make something attractive, you're more likely to *try* doing it. But when you make something satisfying, you're more likely to want more of it, and so you'll *keep coming back* to it. For example, if you replace your afternoon snack of potato chips with snacking on sea salt popcorn instead and you discover that you are really satisfied with the taste of that popcorn, then you're more likely to maintain that snack replacement. The same might not be said if you try to replace the chips with something you don't enjoy as much, like baked kale chips for example.

Stepping out of old habits and into new habits takes self-discipline and time. Your old habits didn't form overnight, so neither will your new ones. But if you remain mindful of The Four Laws of Behavior Change, you're much more likely to stick with the self-discipline and time needed to make it happen.

Don't make a new habit difficult to achieve.

Organize Your Day Around Your Habits

In the spirit of making the new habits you want to implement as easy as possible to achieve, I'm a huge proponent of making sure your entire day is prepped with activities and circumstances to help!

Let's start with your mornings. What do you need to get your day off on the right foot? Whether that means starting on a happy foot, a motivated foot, or a productive foot, set your morning up to make that happen. As an example, for some people, exercising first thing in the morning is their key to exercising at all, so they put their stationary bike or treadmill right in their bedroom and have their workout clothes already laid out from the night before. That way they'll have no distractions in between waking up and getting their body moving.

Personally, I like to start each morning by renewing my mind and refreshing my soul, and nothing does that better for me than listening to some music or to the Bible on audio as I'm drinking my morning glass of refreshing water. To help make sure I do that, I pre-setup my phone app before I go to bed at night to what I want to listen to the next morning. I then set it beside my bed along with a water bottle (my husband got me a Yeti Rambler® too – keeping my water cool and fresh!) so all I need to do when I wake up is click on my app and sip away.

If your habit changes are more focused on your diet, then consider how your kitchen is set up. If you want to start your morning with a smoothie, then have all your smoothie ingredients right there when you open your fridge and freezer. Or, if you'd like to start your morning with a glass of high energy juice, then have what you need right there to do a quick juicing of your favorite concoction. For me that includes two lemons, a couple big handfuls of spinach, a thumb size of fresh ginger, and one green apple. I actually find the process of cutting the fruits and vegetables stimulating, refreshing, and enjoyable as I'm smelling the aromas and thinking about what these nutritious foods are going to do for my mind and body. I do all those things with intentionality – knowing I'm helping my body, mind, and soul work at their absolute best so that I can be productive and purposeful throughout my day. And having them all there when I open the refrigerator makes the process easier. Also, if you're on the go, prep snacks and meals ahead of time so that you don't have to stop at a drive-thru on the way to and from work or at lunch. Instead, you can just grab what you need right from the fridge, setting yourself up for an easy success. So, keeping your fridge and pantry stocked with healthy and satisfying food and doing some meal prep ahead of time are a couple of good ways to organize your day to help you hone and maintain your new healthy eating habit.

Maybe you're a person who prefers working out in the afternoons or evenings rather than first thing in the morning. No problem! You'll find it so helpful to switch gears in the middle of your day and do some exercising if you have workout clothes and equipment that you love to wear and use. Trust me! If you feel satisfaction when you slip into your favorite pair of shorts or leggings, or you love the way your new running sneakers look, or you have an enticing new workout series you've been dying to try, make them readily available and accessible, and you won't be able to talk yourself out of skipping your workout that day. Instead, you'll have created a feeling of energy and a sense of excitement about the activity ahead.

When it comes to winding down at the end of the day and getting yourself ready not only for a good night's sleep, but also for the new day to come, take a close look at your bedroom. Does it create an environment that relaxes you? Have you removed all blue-light screens from the room so your brain can produce the melatonin needed to wind your body down? Is your bed as comfortable and supportive as it needs to be for your sleeping preferences? Have you set up your bedside table for all the items you need to start another great day first thing in the morning? Have you laid your clothes out – whether they're workout clothes, your business outfit, or your favorite mom jeans – so that you don't have to fret and frazzle about making that decision in the morning? There are so many ways you can prep and organize your bedroom to make the following day as habitually productive as possible.

The beauty of setting yourself and your environment up in a way for your habits to thrive is just that: Eventually, you will establish a rhythm for each and every part of your day that you won't be able to skip or ignore your new healthy habit. Your body and mind will come to expect those morning, afternoon, and evening rhythms, giving a place for your new habits to really shine and take hold.

Reflect, Refine, and Renew

Throughout this ongoing process of developing new habits to replace old ones, always remember to reflect on how you're progressing. We've previously discussed how goals are measurable, but sometimes, habits can be harder to measure because they're so automatic. So, a great way to reflect on them is to write about them. At the end of each day, open a fresh page of your journal and write down all the activities you did throughout your day, whether good or bad. Over time, you should start to see patterns forming in those reflections.

From there, you can refine your patterns as needed. For example, if you notice that you don't hydrate nearly enough on the days when you don't prepare a big glass of water to drink first thing in the morning, you'll have the data you need to refine that pattern. Then you can be more deliberate about making the little changes you need to keep progressing.

This is a process and a journey. Stay positive.

Reviewing and refining your habits is what will continuously re-motivate you to keep going with them. Throughout it all, keep remembering your *why,* give yourself grace when you might find you need a break, and renew your mind with your own core beliefs when you need clarity. You might also consider asking your spouse, friend, or your health coach to help keep you accountable - asking them to check in with you each week to give you that extra push to stick with it and to cheerlead you on. This is a process and a journey. Stay positive. *Each time you catch a glimpse of your progress, celebrate and bask in the freshness and health your amazing mind, body, and spirit are experiencing! That is how you will truly hone your healthy habits.*

Action Points: Hone Your Healthy Habits	
Mindset	• Everything you've learned in this book can be implemented or improved by working on the habits associated with them. • Healthy habits aren't necessarily about the end result—learn to fall in love with the process, and you'll love the journey at every step. • Habits are not formed overnight – this is a journey and a process. • There is no "removing bad habits." Only replacing them with good ones. • Grace always
Skillset	• Understand and implement The Four Laws of Behavior Change when planning your new habits. • Make sure your core values, beliefs, wants, and needs fuel the habits you set out to change. • Organize your day and your environment in a way that makes your habits easier to implement.

Action Points:* *Hone Your Healthy Habits	
Toolset	• Your journal is your biggest tool here: Use it to reflect on the habits you have, plan the habits you want to replace them, and the progress you're making toward that goal. • Ask your spouse, friend, or your health coach to help keep you accountable – ask them to check in weekly with you to give you that extra push in an encouraging way. • The additional tools you will use are dependent upon the habits you're trying to form. This book itself is full of ideas for tools to use to form healthy habits, so keep it as an essential tool itself!

Now you are on your way to creating a step-by-step plan for better habits that will lead you to *thriving* health and wellbeing, not for days or weeks, but for a lifetime! My deepest hope is that these habits become your way of living, internalizing them as they automatically become, first and foremost, who you are, not just what you do.

The research I've done for this book draws on biblical insight, as well as biology, neuroscience, and psychology from incredible scientists and doctors. Some of the concepts are long-established, while some are newer and add fresh, exciting layers to the insight, knowledge, and wisdom that has been around for a long time.

Know that you are fully equipped to nurture, support, and strengthen your body, mind, and spirit in the best possible ways. You are a spectacular gift to this world, your loving family, your neighbors, your co-workers, and your community. We need your good and beautiful soul, your giftedness, your convictions, and your strengths. Let's fully invest our one precious life and talents with sustainable enduring vitality for our children, our grandchildren, our community, and our world.

As you continue on this incredible journey, fueled by your core beliefs, may you find deeper joy than you could ever imagine – living *strong, sane, and sassy* in every season of your life as you…

Sense your Body's Signals
Train Your Thought Patterns
Rest and Rejuvenate
Exercise and Move
Nutrify and Hydrate
Goal-Set with Grace
Thrive in Your Community
Hone Your Healthy Habits

Bibliography

Adams, Don, trans. 2017. *Apology by Plato: A New Translation of Plato's Defense of Socrates.* Don Adams.

AdventHealth. "Rest vs. Sleep: Know the Difference for Whole Health," September 21, 2021. https://www.adventhealth.com/blog/rest-vs-sleep-know-difference-whole-health. Accessed May 9, 2023

American Osteopathic Association. "The Benefits of Yoga," n.d. https://osteopathic.org/what-is-osteopathic-medicine/benefits-of-yoga/. Accessed May 5, 2023

Andrews, Maria. "Does Running Help You Live Longer? The Life-Extending Benefits of Running." *Marathonhandbook.Com,* November 18, 2022. https://marathonhandbook.com/does-running-help-you-live-longer/#:~:text=The%20collective%20data%20from%20all,of%20death%20from%20all%20cancers%20.

Bond, Michael. 2017. "Ready for Anything: The Best Strategies to Survive a Disaster." *New Scientist,* May 10, 2017. https://www.newscientist.com/article/mg23431250-400-ready-for-anything-the-best-strategy-to-survive-a-disaster/. Accessed May 5, 2023.

Crossway Bibles. T*he ESV Study Bible: English Standard Version.* Wheaton, IL: Crossway Bibles, 2001.

Clear, James. *Atomic Habits: An Easy and Proven Way to Build Good Habits and Break Bad Ones.* New York, NY: Avery, 2018.

Elliot, Brianna. "Epsom Salt: Benefits, Uses, and Side Effects." *Healthline.Com,* February 21, 2023. https://www.healthline.com/nutrition/epsom-salt-benefits-uses#benefits.

Elliot Physical Therapy. "The Importance Of Proper Breathing For Your Overall Health," September 26, 2017. https://elliott-physicaltherapy.com/importance-proper-breathing-overall-health/. Accessed May 7, 2023.

Epel, Elissa, Jennifer Daubenmier, Judith Tedlie Moskowitz, Susan Folkman, and Elizabeth Blackburn. "Can Meditation Slow Rate of Cellular Aging? Cognitive Stress, Mindfulness, and Telomeres." *Annals of the New York Academy of Sciences* 1172, no. 1 (August 2009): 34–53. https://doi.org/10.1111/j.1749-6632.2009.04414.x.

Fuhrman, Joel. *Eat to Live: The Amazing Nutrient-Rich Program for Fast and Sustained Weight Loss,* Revised Edition. Boston, MA: Little, Brown Spark, 2011.

Groth, Leah. "Can You Lose Weight by Drinking Water?" *Everydayhealth.Com,* May 10, 2021. https://www.everyday-health.com/weight/can-you-lose-weight-by-drinking-water/.

Harvard Health Publishing. "Foods Linked to Better Brain-power," March 6, 2021. https://www.health.harvard.edu/health-beat/foods-linked-to-better-brainpower. Accessed May 6, 2023.

Harvard School of Public Health - The Nutrition Source. "Omega-3 Fatty Acids: An Essential Contribution," September 18, 2012. https://www.hsph.harvard.edu/nutritionsource/what-should-you-eat/fats-and-cholesterol/types-of-fat/omega-3-fats/. Accessed May 6, 2023.

Harvard School of Public Health - The Nutrition Source. "Vegetables and Fruits," September 18, 2012. https://www.hsph.harvard.edu/nutritionsource/what-should-you-eat/vegetables-and-fruits/. Accessed May 6, 2023.

Hyatt, Michael. "5 Reasons Why You Should Commit Your Goals to Writing." Fullfocus.Co, October 20, 2022. https://fullfocus.co/5-reasons-why-you-should-commit-your-goals-to-writing/#:~:text=The%20research%20is%20conclusive.,just%20by%20writing%20them%20down.

Inc. Staff. 1611 Edition KJV Bible. Peabody, MA: Hendrickson Publishers, 2003.

Integris Health. "Why It's Important to Allow Yourself to Rest," April 16, 2021. https://integrisok.com/resources/on-your-health/2021/april/why-its-important-to-allow-yourself-to-rest. Accessed May 5, 2023.

Kosslynn, Stephan and Thompson, William. The Neural Basis of Mental Imagery. MIT Press, 2006.

Li, William W. Eat to Beat Disease: The New Science of How Your Body Can Heal Itself. New York, NY: Balance, 2019.

Mineo, Liz. "Good Genes Are Nice, but Joy Is Better." News.Harvard.Edu. April 11, 2017. https://news.harvard.edu/gazette/story/2017/04/over-nearly-80-years-harvard-study-has-been-showing-how-to-live-a-healthy-and-happy-life/.

Morrison, Leesa. "Let Food Be Thy Medicine," December 27, 2015. https://theghoshcircle.org/blog/let-food-be-thy-medicine. Accessed May 6, 2023.

Newberry, Tommy. Success Is Not an Accident: Change Your Choices; Change Your Life. Carol Stream, IL: Tyndale House Publishers, 2007.

Newberry, Tommy. The 4:8 Principle: The Secret to a Joy-Filled Life. Carol Stream, IL: Tyndale House Publishers, 2007.

NIH - National Institute of General Medical Sciences (NIGMS). "National Institute of General Medical Sciences – Circadian Rhythms," n.d.
https://nigms.nih.gov/education/fact-sheets/Pages/circadian-rhythms.aspx#:~:text=%E2%80%8B%E2%80%8BWhat%20are%20circadian,the%20study%20of%20circadian%20rhythms. Accessed May 5, 2023.

Ornish, Dean, and Anne Ornish. *Undo It!: How Simple Lifestyle Changes Can Reverse Most Chronic Diseases.* New York, NY: Ballantine Books, 2019.

Oura. "Why Sleep Matters," March 10, 2023.
https://ouraring.com/blog/why-does-sleep-matter/.
Accessed May 10, 2023.

Oxford Languages. "Neuroplasticity." In *Google.Com.*
Accessed May 5, 2023.
https://www.google.com/search?rlz=1C1CHBF_enUS932US932&sxsrf=APwXEdf8FVHrZkFIG5BHkadTTJtNRrQUA:1683321773900&q=neuroplasticity&si=AMnBZoE_SgVdNzFvWI74rwHkJYEE_WKpG0HwqsHc4Zu7FlHHMonW6qvH4NSdGqXB_azTw28cSHa0RL2dKJitQGeVeSc-JJiic-_WGTCdo9AXJO-HOwLVesho%3D&expnd=1&sa=X&ved=2ahUKEwjL14Cjjt_-AhVfiO4BHaAMCAUQ2v4IegQICRAR&biw=1280&bih=569&dpr=1.5.

Oxford Population Health – Cancer Epidemiology Unit (CEU). "Study of Almost 400,000 Confirms That Higher Blood Levels of IGF-1 Are a Risk Factor for Several Types of Cancer." September 15, 2020. https://www.ceu.ox.ac.uk/news/study-of-almost-400-000-confirms-that-higher-blood-levels-of-igf-1-are-a-risk-factor-for-several-types-of-cancer. Accessed May 6, 2023.

Ram, Kaushik. 2022. "How Does the Brain Tell the Real from Imagined? – TEDxSydney." n.d. https://tedxsydney.com/idea/how-does-the-brain-tell-the-real-from-imagined/. Accessed May 4, 2023.

Schwartz, Tony. "Relax! You'll Be More Productive!" *Nytimes.Com.* February 9, 2013. https://www.nytimes.com/2013/02/10/opinion/sunday/relax-youll-be-more-productive.html.

SCL Health. 2018. "The Power of Hugs and How They Affect Our Daily Health," n.d. https://www.sclhealth.org/blog/2019/07/the-power-of-hugs-and-how-they-affect-our-daily-health/. Accessed May 5, 2023.

Selfpause. "The Science Behind Visualization and Muscle Growth: A Study." 2023. https://selfpause.com/visualization/visualization-and-muscle-growth/. Accessed May 4, 2023.

Shinn, Florence Scovel. *The Collected Wisdom of Florence Scovel Shinn: The Game of Life and How to Play It: Your Word Is Your Wand, the Secret Door to Success, the Power of the Spoken Word.* San Diego, CA: The Book Tree, 2010.

Thames, Brenda J. and Deborah J. Thomason. 1997. "NASD - Stress Management for the Health of It." n.d. https://nasdonline.org/1445/d001245/stress-management-for-the-health-of-it.html Accessed May 5, 2023.

Waldinger, Robert J., Shiri Cohen, Marc S. Schulz, and Judith A. Crowell. "Security of Attachment to Spouses in Late Life: Concurrent And Prospective Links with Cognitive and Emotional Wellbeing." PubMed Central (PMC), August 18, 2014. https://doi.org/10.1177/2167702614541261. Accessed May 8, 2023.

Suggested Reading

Here is a list of books from my personal library that I highly recommend reading to further your journey to authentic health and lasting wellness!

English Standard Version (ESV) Bible. Crossway, 2001.

Anatomy Of The Soul by Curt Thompson, M.D. Tyndale House Publishers, Inc., 2010.

Atomic Habits: An Easy and Proven Way to Build Good Habits and Break Bad Ones by James Clear. Avery, 2018.

Bone Broth Diet by Kellyann Petrucci, MS, ND. Rodale, 2015.

Boundaries For Your Soul: How To Turn Your Overwhelming Thoughts And Feelings Into Your Greatest Allies by Alison Cook Ph.D. and Kimberly Miller MTb LMFT. Thomas Nelson, 2018.

Eat to Beat Disease: The New Science of How Your Body Can Heal Itself by William W. Li. Balance, 2019.

Emotionally Healthy Spirituality by Peter Scazzero. Zondervan, 2006.

Free Of Me: Why Life Is Better When It's Not About You by Sharon Hodde Miller. Baker Books, 2017.

Goals! How To Get Everything You Want – Faster Than You Ever Thought Possible by Brian Tracy. MJF Books, 2010.

How To Heal Your Metabolism: Stop Blaming Aging For Your Slowing Metabolism by Kate Deering. Createspace Independent Publishing Platform, 2015.

Inner Excellence: Train Your Mind For Extraordinary Performance And The Best Possible Life by Jim Murphy. Published by the Academy of Excellence, 2020.

Love Your Gut: Supercharge Your Digestive Health And Transform Your Well Being From The Inside Out by Dr. Megan Rossi. Dreamscape Media, 2021.

Metabolical: The Lure And The Lies Of Processed Food, Nutrition, And Modern Medicine by Robert H Lustig MD MSL. Harper Wave, 2021.

Success Is Not An Accident: Change Your Choices, Change Your Life by Tommy Newberry. Tyndale House Publishers, Inc., 2007.

Super Immunity: The Essential Guide For boosting Your Body's Defenses To Live Longer, Stronger, And Disease Free by Joel Furhman, MD. HarperOne, 2013.

Switch On Your Brain: The Key To Peak Happiness, Thinking, And Health by Dr. Caroline Leaf. Baker Books, 2013.

The 4:8 Principle: The Secret To A Joy-Filled Life by Tommy Newberry. Tyndale House Publishers, Inc., 2007.

The Best Of You: Break Free From Painful Patterns, Mend Your Past, & Discover Your True Self In God by Dr. Alison Cook. Thomas Nelson, 2023.

The Choice: Embrace The Possible by Dr. Edith Eva Eger. Scribner, 2017.

The Gifts Of Imperfection: Let Go Of Who You Think You're Supposed To Be And Embrace Who You Are: Your Guide To A Wholehearted Life by Brené Brown, Ph. D. Hazelden, 2010.

The Gut-Immune Connection: How Understanding The Connection Between Food And Immunity Can Help Us Regain Our Health by Emeran Mayer MD. Harper Wave, 2021.

The Immune System Recovery Plan: A Doctor's 4-Step Plan: Achieve Optimal Health And Feel Your Best, Strengthen Your Immune System, Treat Autoimmune Disease by Susan Blum, MD, MPH. Scribner Book Company, 2013.

The Molecular Nutrition Of Amino Acids And Proteins by Dominique Dardevet. Academic Press, 2016.

The Purpose Driven Life: What On Earth Am I Here For? by Rick Warren. Zondervan, 2002.

The Soul Of Shame by Curt Thompson, M.D. InterVarsity Press, Inc., 2015.

The Well Regulated Nervous System: A Nervous System Workbook & Journal by Kelsey Rising. Independently published, 2023.

Think & Eat Yourself Smart: A Neuroscientific Approach To A Sharper Mind and Healthier Life by Dr. Caroline Leaf. Baker Books, 2016.

Think, Learn, Succeed: Understanding And Using Your Mind To Thrive At School, The Workplace, And Life by Dr. Caroline Leaf. Baker Books, 2018.

Think Like A Winner! by Dr. Walter Doyle Staples. Melvin Powers Wilshire Book Company, 1991.

Thinking For A Change: 11 Ways Highly Successful People Approach Life And Work by John C. Maxwell. Center Street, 2003.

Who Switched Off My Brain? Controlling Toxic Thoughts And Emotions by Dr. Caroline Leaf. Thomas Nelson Publishers, 2009.

Undo It! How Simple Lifestyle Changes Can Reverse Most Chronic Diseases by Dean and Anne Ornish. Ballantine Books, 2019.

Acknowledgments

Writing a book is harder than I ever thought, and more rewarding than I could have ever imagined. None of this would have been possible without the love and support from my family and friends. André, your unwavering devotion, strength, and stability provided a strong foundation for me throughout the journey of writing this book. You believed in me when my own doubt and fear threatened to hold me back. I still find it hard to believe that you are mine and grateful that we are always on each other's team.

To my three loving children, Charisse, Michael, and Rachelle, and to their remarkable spouses, Joel, Rachel, and Noah: You are a fountain of inspiration and motivation to me as I watch you build your lives and family with great faith, heart, and truth. The love I hold for each of you defies expression on paper; it resides deep within my heart.

To my eight indescribably beautiful grandchildren, your unique gifts, personalities, and strengths leave me in awe and gratitude. You are my greatest treasure, and every moment spent with you lights up my life. Your radiant spark takes my breath away.

I want to express my heartfelt gratitude to my fiercely loving and faithful friends. Thank you for challenging me, laughing with me, crying with me, and praying with me season after season. Whether I was residing in Virginia, Ohio, Florida, California, or Georgia, your presence in my life has been an anchor.

To Beth and Dan, Jackie, Mary, Karla and Dave, Heidi, Kim, Linda, Lynn, Debra, Alice, Jess, Brenda, Kristen, Laura, Dena, Tamazeen, Phyllis, Andrea, Julie, Mara, Deby, Anne, Jeannie, Cindy, Karen, Jodie, Sonja, Michelle, Becky, Christine, Karen, Terri, my Uncle RT, Janet, Stephanie, Dayna, the members of my yoga training class, the exceptional teaching staff and Cru staff at "the" Ohio State University, and countless others, please know that I hold your deposits into my life close to my heart. Your love and support have helped shape me into the person I am today.

To my publisher, editors, and book cover designer, your skills, expertise, and patience with me went far beyond my expectations. Thank you!

I am profoundly grateful to my parents, Richard and Jane, for their enduring love, guidance, and influence.

Ultimately, my deepest gratitude goes to God – the one who knows me fully and loves me unconditionally. God, who created me, leads me, rescues me, sustains me, and grants me each precious breath. The joy and fulfillment I experience are beyond measure, and I am humbled by His boundless love and grace.

This book is a testament to the profound impact of the people who have truly known me and loved me. Thank you from the depths of my heart.

With love and gratitude,

Lynda Hébert